Case-Based
Medical Physiology

Case-Based Medical Physiology

Professor Christopher Bell PhD, DSc, FTCD

Department of Physiology
The University of Dublin
Faculty of Health Sciences
Trinity College Dublin
Dublin
Ireland

Professor Emeritus Cecil Kidd PhD, FIBiol, FRSA

School of Medical Sciences
College of Life Sciences & Medicine
University of Aberdeen
Aberdeen
Scotland

Professor Trefor Morgan MD, FRACP

Department of Physiology
University of Melbourne
Victoria
Australia

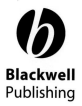

Blackwell
Publishing

© 2005 C. Bell, C. Kidd, T. Morgan.
Published by Blackwell Publishing Ltd

Blackwell Publishing, Inc., 350 Main Street, Malden, Massachusetts 02148–5020, USA
Blackwell Publishing Ltd, 9600 Garsington Road, Oxford OX4 2DQ, UK
Blackwell Publishing Asia Pty Ltd, 550 Swanston Street, Carlton, Victoria 3053, Australia

First published 2005

Library of Congress Cataloging-in-Publication Data
Bell, Christopher, 1941-
 Case-based medical physiology / Christopher Bell, Cecil Kidd, Trefor Morgan.
  p. ; cm.
Includes bibliographical references index.
ISBN-13: 978-1-4051-2061-6
ISBN-10: 1-4051-2061-4
1. Physiology, Pathological--Case studies.
[DNLM: 1. Clinical Medicine--Case Reports. 2. Clinical Medicine--Problems and Exercises. 3. Diagnosis, Differential--Case Reports. 4. Diagnosis, Differential--Problems and Exercises. 5. Physiological Processes--Case Reports. 6. Physiological Processes--Problems and Exercises. 7. Signs and Symptoms--Case Reports. 8. Signs and Symptoms--Problems and Exercises. 9. Therapeutics--Case Reports. 10. Therapeutics--Problems and Exercises.
] I. Kidd, C. (Cecil), 1933- II. Morgan, Trefor O. III. Title.
RB113.B445 2005
616.07'5--dc22

                                                           2005003365

ISBN-13: 978-1-4051-20616
ISBN-10: 1-4051-20614

A catalogue record for this title is available from the British Library
Set in 10/12 pt Minion by Sparks, Oxford – www.sparks.co.uk

Printed and bound in India by Replika Press PVT Ltd.

Commissioning Editor: Vicki Noyes
Development Editor: Geraldine Jeffers
Production Controller: Kate Charman

For further information on Blackwell Publishing, visit our website:
http://www.blackwellpublishing.com

Contents

Preface

Our aim in writing this book of case studies has been to provide a new approach to clinical physiology, distinct from the standard texts that either concentrate on basic human physiology or focus on clinical presentation and treatment. The book is intended for medical students in both 'problem-solving' and more traditional curricula, and should also be useful to students at an advanced stage of courses in paramedical and biomedical sciences.

The cases highlight the physiological basis of some situations that are met with fairly commonly in clinical practice. They have intentionally not been grouped according to body system, since our emphasis is on how multiple systems interact in real life. Nonetheless, the index allows you to locate all cases dealing with specific systems, if you wish.

Each case is accompanied by multiple-choice questions in the formats used in many undergraduate and postgraduate programmes, including the USMLE. There are answers and feedback for each question, some open questions that ask you to think about particular aspects of the case and some suggestions for additional specialist reading. We avoid recommending a specific textbook of medical physiology for background reading, because of the variety used in different medical schools: any of the commonly prescribed texts contains appropriate material.

Most of the cases involve questions about numerical variables with which any medical graduate should be familiar. As guidance, we have given what we consider typical normal values for these variables in the Western world, based on our experience and on the consensus of published material. Slightly different values will be found in some textbooks and in some populations but the variations should not be sufficient to cause confusion.

Our aim has been to discuss the physiological basis for diagnosis and treatment, not to provide definitive answers on clinical management. Thus, although we have tried to ensure that all information is clinically accurate, situations have sometimes been simplified. For instance, on occasions only a limited number of possibilities are discussed when a wider range of options would need to be considered in practice. For full authoritative information on diagnosis and management, you should consult your clinical teachers.

A number of colleagues have provided useful input by commenting on aspects of chapter content and supplying illustrative material. In particular, thanks are due to Dr Conal Cunningham, Mr Bernard Donne, Dr Mary Keogan, Dr Patrick Manning, Dr Niall Mulvihill, Dr Paul Tierney and Professor Michael Walsh.

C.B.
C.K.
T.O.M.

Neck injury from a swimming accident

CASE AND MCQS

Case introduction

Sean W. is a 22-year-old college graduate from Seattle. To celebrate his graduation, he and some friends are taking a camping holiday in Queensland, Australia. One morning they are swimming in an estuary and Sean dives into the water, unaware that there is a sandbank just a metre below the surface. He floats to the surface a couple of seconds later, semi-conscious and unable to move. His friends are able to roll him onto a surfboard and carry him to the shore.

He is conscious and breathing, but his arms and legs are limp and he says that he cannot feel anything in his body or move his limbs. His friends ring the emergency services and tell the operator that Sean has probably broken his neck.

Q1 If Sean is breathing spontaneously, this indicates that the connections of his brain to the spinal nerves *must* be intact as far caudal as:

A. nerve C_2
B. nerve C_5
C. nerve C_6
D. nerve C_7
E. nerve C_8

Q2 If intact neural function was preserved to this segmental level, the most rostral point at which vertebral damage can have occurred is:

A. between C_4 and C_5 vertebrae
B. between C_5 and C_6 vertebrae
C. between C_6 and C_7 vertebrae
D. between C_7 and C_8 vertebrae
E. none of the above

On arrival, the paramedics immobilize Sean's head and spine with an inflatable collar and a Kendrick jacket, so as to prevent further damage at the trauma site. Then they check his blood pressure and heart rate.

Q3 Given the site of the spinal lesion you would predict that, relative to a normal individual lying supine, there would be:

A. high blood pressure and low heart rate
B. high blood pressure and high heart rate
C. low blood pressure and low heart rate
D. low blood pressure and high heart rate
E. no change from normal

Sean is transported to the nearest hospital with a spinal unit. Before he is sent to the radiology department for X-ray, the neurologist carries out cutaneous sensory tests to help establish the severity and level of the lesion. He finds that Sean has normal touch sensation over his shoulders, the lateral half of his arms, thumb and first fingers, but cannot feel touch or pinprick along the inner margin of his arms, the centre of his palms or the middle, ring or little fingers (Fig. 1.1).

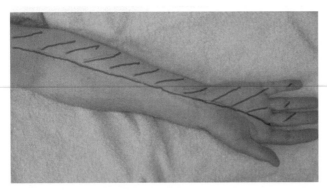

Fig. 1.1 Sean's right arm as marked by the neurologist. The pen marks show the area of sensory loss.

Q4 This distribution of anaesthesia indicates that the *most caudal* intact spinal nerve is:

A. C_5
B. C_6
C. C_7
D. C_8
E. T_1

The site of lesion is confirmed by radiology. Initial X-ray does not yield a clear image because of interference from the shoulder bones, but subsequent MRI clearly indicates dislocation of C_6 and C_7 vertebrae, with compression of the spinal cord (Fig. 1.2).

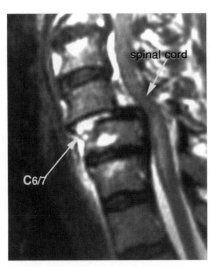

Fig. 1.2 Lateral T_2-weighted MRI image of Sean's neck, showing dislocation of C_6 and C_7 vertebrae.

Q5 With a spinal lesion at this level, which of the following ocular functions would be *abnormal*?

A. blinking in response to corneal irritation
B. tear secretion
C. resting level of the upper eyelid
D. both A and B
E. all of A, B and C

Q6 With a spinal lesion at this level, which of the following circulatory reflexes would be *abnormal*?

A. bradycardia in response to left ventricular baroreceptor activation
B. bradycardia in response to carotid arterial baroreceptor activation
C. bradycardia in response to aortic arch baroreceptor activation
D. all of the above
E. none of the above

Q7 With a spinal lesion at this level, which of the following respiratory functions would be *normal*?

A. bronchiolar mucus clearance
B. bronchiolar mucus secretion
C. Forced vital capacity
D. both A and B
E. all of A, B and C

Q8 With a spinal lesion at this level, which of the following upper digestive tract functions would be *normal*?

A. salivation
B. swallowing
C. duodenal secretion of gastrin
D. gastric receptive relaxation
E. all of the above

Q9 With a spinal lesion at this level, which of the following lower digestive tract functions would be *abnormal*?

A. gastro-colic reflex in response to food in the stomach
B. ileocaecal sphincter opening in response to ileal filling
C. jejunal peristalsis during food digestion
D. defaecation
E. both A and D

Q10 With a spinal lesion at this level, which of the following endocrine functions would be *abnormal*?

A. aldosterone release in response to reduced plasma potassium
B. vasopressin release in response to increased plasma osmolality
C. adrenaline release in response to reduced plasma volume
D. insulin release in response to reduced plasma glucose
E. none of the above

Q11 With a spinal lesion at this level, which of the following motor functions would be *normal*?

A. wrist extension
B. wrist flexion
C. elbow extension
D. finger flexion
E. all of the above

Because of the prolonged immobility, thromboembolism is a major concern over the first few weeks after spinal injury. For this reason, anticoagulants are given routinely as soon as any risk of haemorrhage has gone. The standard drug of choice for early treatment is heparin, administered by injection twice daily.

Q12 Heparin acts as an anticoagulant by:

A. catalysing breakdown of fibrin
B. catalysing binding of thrombin to antithrombin
C. inhibiting binding of fibrin to platelets
D. inhibiting activation of tisue thromboplastin
E. inhibiting activation of factor VII

Q13 Physiologically, heparin is thought to serve a role in preventing inappropriate clotting. The heparin molecule is located:

A. in mast cells
B. in neutrophils
C. in endothelial cells
D. at all of the above sites
E. at none of the above sites

Heparin has a rapid onset of action, but for long-term use there is the practical problem that it has to be injected as it is not absorbed through the intestinal mucosa. Prolonged anticoagulant treatment needs a drug that can be given orally so, after anticoagulation is established with heparin, it is replaced by an orally active coumarin molecule such as warfarin. These agents are not suitable for acute treatment because they have a delayed onset of action, with anticoagulant activity not beginning for about 12 hours and becoming more pronounced over the next 2 days.

Q14 Coumarin anticoagulants have a long latency of action because:

A. their absorption from the gut is very slow
B. they act by inactivating clotting factors that have half-lives of up to 30 hours
C. they act by binding to platelets that have a half-life of about 30 hours
D. their action depends on enzymic conversion into an active molecule
E. their action depends on synthesis of new vitamin K in the liver

Because Sean's bladder is paralysed immediately after his accident, he has a urethral catheter inserted into the bladder that allows continual passage of urine. After a month, however, clinical assessment suggests that his sacral spinal reflexes have become active enough to allow reflex micturition to take place.

Q15 Micturition controlled by spinal reflex pathways will differ from that in intact individuals in the following way(s):

A. there is automatic voiding when bladder filling reaches a critical volume
B. there is activation of voiding by cutaneous mechanoreceptor stimulation
C. no voiding occurs even with a full bladder without cutaneous mechanoreceptor stimulation
D. both A and B
E. both B and C

One of the concerns in patients with spinal paralysis is that their bladders do not empty as completely as normal, and the retained urine sometimes becomes a site of infection.

Q16 Effective strategies for reducing the risk of urinary tract infections include:

A. routine oral antibiotics
B. routine ingestion of agents that will make the urine more alkaline
C. routine ingestion of large volumes of fluid
D. restriction of dietary protein
E. none of the above

Because of the absence of sensory connections from his bladder, Sean is unable to feel that his bladder is full. However, he notices that, shortly before it reaches the volume that triggers automatic voiding, his face starts to feel hot. This is useful because it helps him to have voluntary control over a function that would otherwise occur unpredictably.

Q17 The reason for Sean's face feeling hot when his bladder is distended is:

A. spinal reflex activation of sympathetic vasoconstrictor nerves above the lesion
B. spinal reflex inhibition of sympathetic vasoconstrictor nerves above the lesion
C. spinal reflex activation of sympathetic vasoconstrictor nerves below the lesion
D. spinal reflex inhibition of sympathetic vasoconstrictor nerves below the lesion
E. spinal reflex inhibition of sweating above the lesion

The principles that we have just looked at in relation to urinary tract function also apply to defaecation. Once again, there is no direct awareness of visceral distension and automatic sacral reflex voiding occurs. As with bladder function, it is possible to detect imminent voiding by sympathetic dysreflexia and also possible to trigger the voiding volitionally by stimulating skin mechanoreceptors.

However, it is not possible to void faeces into a bag like urine. Coping with defaecation can therefore be a considerable burden to the spinal patient. To simplify matters, most paraplegics aim to regulate their bowel activity so they pass stools only once every 2 days.

With this relatively long interval, dietary patterns need to be carefully tailored so as to avoid constipation.

Q18 Strategies for preventing constipation include:

A. reducing colonic water reabsorption
B. increasing growth of colonic bacteria
C. shortening colonic transit time
D. increasing intracolonic osmolality
E. all of the above

Over the first few weeks after injury, the muscles in Sean's legs show a tendency to contract spontaneously, resulting in maintained flexion of his hips and knees.

Q19 Spasticity in the limbs below a spinal lesion is caused by:

A. degeneration of damaged motor nerves
B. regeneration of damaged motor nerves
C. degeneration of denervated muscle fibres
D. development of spontaneous activity in spinal motor neurons
E. loss of descending inhibitory effects on spinal motor neurons

As Sean becomes used to his situation, he is able to begin to train himself to become more mobile and self-sufficient and to think about his future. One recurring problem is the fact that every time he transfers from bed to wheelchair he feels faint, with blurred vision and ringing in his ears.

Q20 These symptoms occurring with postural change are caused by:

A. reduced blood pressure secondary to redistribution of regional perfusion
B. reduced blood pressure secondary to venous pooling
C. reduced cerebral perfusion secondary to autoregulation
D. increased blood pressure secondary to sympathetic dysreflexia
E. increased cerebral perfusion secondary to autoregulation

Q21 This problem could be reduced by:

A. elevating plasma levels of vasopressin (ADH) by water restriction
B. elevating plasma levels of angiotensin by sodium restriction
C. mechanical venous compression
D. elevating plasma levels of adrenaline (epinephrine) by regular glucose ingestion
E. all of A, B and C

Sean plans to live at home and is worried about the special facilities that will be needed. Also, he and his girlfriend want to know whether they will be able to have children.

Q22 Consider the impact of Sean's injury on his motor system. In planning the home facilities that he needs, it has to be borne in mind that he:

A. will not be able to type without a mouth control
B. will need to use his shoulders or a mouth control to switch on lights
C. will need a wrist support in order to be able to clean his teeth
D. will not be able to assist with dressing himself
E. all of the above

Q23 In counselling Sean it is important to remember that his capacity to father children will be limited by the fact that:

A. his sperm count will be reduced because of scrotal vaso-dilation
B. his semen volume will be reduced because of prostate denervation
C. his ejaculatory capacity will be reduced because of reflux into the bladder
D. his erectile capacity will be reduced because of absent corticospinal drive
E. all of the above

Q24 If an injury similar to Sean's had happened to a young woman, what implications would there be for her sexuality and her capacity to become a mother?

Consider the overall physiological consequences of Sean's situation. In this case study we have identified a number of specific functions that will be disrupted, some mainly in the acute post-injury phase and some permanent.

Q25 What other long-term physiological problems do you think need to be considered when planning his lifestyle and in designing a suitable rehabilitation programme?

MCQ ANSWERS AND FEEDBACK

1.B. Motor roots supplying the phrenic nerve exit via C_3–C_5 spinal roots, so damage at the C_2 level would prevent activation of all respiratory muscles. The intercostal muscles are supplied by thoracic spinal nerves and will be inactive after cervical section at any segment, but diaphragmatic activity alone is sufficient to provide adequate resting ventilation.

2.A. Remember that the most rostral spinal nerve (C_1) exits between the occiput of the skull and the atlas (C_1 vertebra). Therefore, each of the more caudal segmental nerves must exit *above* its correspondingly numbered vertebra.

3.D. Removal of the descending drive from the hindbrain cardiovascular control centre to thoracolumbar sympathetic preganglionic neurons will cause a profound fall in total peripheral resistance and reduce blood pressure. However, both the sensory and vagal motor components of the arterial baroreflex pathway are intact, as they are cranial nerves, so the hypotension will cause tachycardia via reflex reduction in vagal cardiac tone.

4.B. Typical cutaneous distributions of the lower cervical nerves are:

- C_5 lateral margin of arm
- C_6 central area of arm, lateral wrist, thumb, first finger
- C_7 central area wrist and palm, middle finger
- C_8 medial area wrist and palm, fourth and little fingers.

There is some individual variability, however, in the distribution of C_6–C_8 between different fingers. The medial surface of the arm above mid-forearm level receives its sensory innervation from thoracic nerves.

5.C. Cervical cord section will remove all connections between the brain and sympathetic outflows, including that to the levator palpebrae muscles, which originates from T_{1-2} spinal nerves and travels to the head via the cervical sympathetic trunk. By contrast, the somatic reflex mediating blinking and the parasympathetic reflex mediating lacrimation involve only cranial pathways and so are undamaged.

6.E. The reflex arc coupling baroreceptor inputs and vagal cardiac control involves only cranial nerves. By contrast, baroreflex responses involving sympathetic outflows (needed for vasoconstriction and for tachycardia above about 110 beats/min) are abolished after cervical section.

7.B. Mucus secretion is regulated by cranial neural activity via the vagus. If the intercostal musculature is paralysed, both mucus clearance from the airways by coughing and the absolute extent to which the thorax can expand and contract will be reduced.

8.E. Salivary secretion is controlled by cranial nerves 7 and 9 (facial and glossopharyngeal). The initiation of swallowing is by somatic cranial impulses to tongue and pharyngeal muscles, and the oesphageal component depends only on enteric peristaltic circuits in the wall of the oesophagus itself. Gastrin secretion from the duodeum is stimulated by entry of protein fragments into that part of the intestine and is independent of neural influences. Both afferent and efferent axons mediating receptive reflex relaxation of the stomach travel in the vagus.

9.D. Defaecation normally involves synchronized contraction of a variety of voluntary muscle groups simultaneously with parasympathetic contraction of the rectal wall. These events are coordinated through the brain. The gastro-colic reflex appears to involve only thoracolumbar spinal reflex circuitry. Small bowel peristalsis during digestion and the passage of chyme from small bowel to caecum are controlled primarily by circulating gastrin levels.

10.C. Stimulation of adrenal medullary secretion in response to lowered plasma volume involves sensory inputs to the hindbrain from low-pressure atrial baroreceptors and descending motor inputs from hindbrain to thoracic preganglionic sympathetic neurons. All the other responses listed involve direct detection of changes in plasma composition by the endocrine cells involved.

11.A. Wrist flexion and finger and elbow extension depend on C_7 and finger flexion is mediated via C_8.

12.B. Circulating antithrombin normally inhibits the activation of several factors (including thrombin) in the intrinsic and common clotting cascades. Antithrombin acts as a 'suicide substrate', with the clotting factor binding to a specific reactive site on the antithrombin molecule and becoming trapped there. In the presence of heparin, the rate of the factor–antithrombin reaction is speeded up around 1000-fold, completely preventing clot formation.

13.A. Heparin is found in mast cells and basophils, although its physiological functions in these cells are not well understood. It is also expressed on the surface of endothelial cells and in the subendothelial cell matrix, where it probably acts to reduce the likelihood of spontaneous clots in response to trivial microcirculatory damage.

14.B. The coumarin agents prevent activation of clotting factors by vitamin K. A number of these factors are vitamin K-dependent and they have turnover times that range from 6 hours (factor VII) to more than 2 days (factor II). This variation means that the anticoagulant effect of coumarins develops progressively over 2–3 days, as more and more steps in the clotting cascade become affected.

15.D. Although there is a sacral reflex pathway between bladder stretch-receptive axons and the parasympathetic motor outflow to the bladder wall, this is normally depressed by descending inhibitory impulses from the brain except during voluntary micturition. If the descending inhibitory influence is removed by spinal damage, stretch receptor activation triggers reflex bladder contraction whenever bladder volume exceeds a critical value – typically around 500–600 ml. Figure 1.3 illustrates the circuitry involved. The autonomic preganglionic neurons also receive excitatory inputs from cutaneous mechanoreceptors but normally these are also overridden by the descending inhibition. In a spinal patient, however, they can be used to initiate reflex micturition by tapping on the pubic wall, pulling the pubic hair or stroking the inner surface of the thighs.

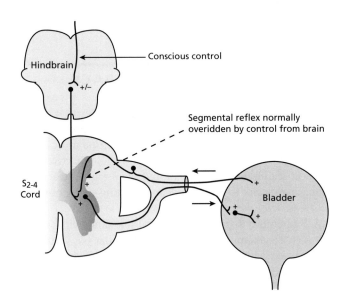

Fig. 1.3 Dual sacral and hindbrain control of the micturition reflex. The (+) and (–) symbols denote sites of excitatory and inhibitory synapses.

16.C. The most efficient protection against urinary tract infection is the acidity of urine, which makes it a poor culture medium for most microorganisms. When there is a high risk of urinary retention, infection can be minimized by ingestion of a filterable organic acid such as ascorbic acid and by a fluid intake of at least 3 litres/day to ensure good bladder flushing. Antibiotic therapy is sometimes required if an infection develops, but continual administration is not necessary and carries the danger of producing bacterial resistance. Protein restriction would reduce total body load of organic acid and so make the urine alkaline.

17.C. Removal of descending inhibition allows reflex activation of preganglionic neurons by a variety of spinal sensory inputs. One of these is the cutaneous mechanoreceptor input onto sacral parasympathetic neurons that we saw in the context of Question 15. In addition, bladder wall stretch-receptive nerves have inputs to thoracolumbar sympathetic neurons. Bladder distension therefore causes reflex vasoconstriction, increasing peripheral resistance and blood pressure. This is a phenomenon termed sympathetic dysreflexia. In facial skin, where sympathetic innervation is not as dense as in some regions, elevated blood pressure produces increased blood flow. Since the sensory innervation of this region is intact, the increased flow is detected as facial warming.

18.E. The most satisfactory approach to prevention and treatment of constipation is a diet rich in non-absorbable vegetable fibre, which represents a mixture of polysaccharides such as cellulose and pectin, plus waxes and glycoproteins. Fibre binds water and ions in the colonic lumen and also supports the growth of colonic bacteria. These contribute further to faecal bulk and increase local water retention by metabolizing some of the fibre molecules and raising intraluminal osmolality. The end result of increased faecal mass is to distend the colon: this initiates peristaltic waves that maintain faecal transit into the rectum.

19.E. This problem has a similar basis to the enhanced autonomic reflex gain discussed in the feedback to Questions 15 and 17. In the intact spinal cord, somatic lower motor neurons are continually under descending inhibitory control from the brain. Once this inhibition is removed, the motor neurons become subject to continual excitatory inputs from sensory sources such as muscle stretch receptors that normally never cause supra-threshold depolarization. Since the muscle contractions lead to more sensory input, sustained contracture results.

Unless limb flexion is prevented by use of drugs or local anaesthesia, there is a danger that this situation will lead to irreversible changes in limb position that seriously limit the patient's capacity to lie down or sit. Also, effective use of prosthetic devices to improve arm and hand movements relies on the limb position being normal. For these reasons it is essential to prevent maintained flexion contractures leading to irreversible structural changes in joints, muscles and tendons. Especially after high spinal injury, the hands should be splinted in a resting position as soon as possible and until the period of lower motor neuron hypersensitivity has passed.

20.B. These symptoms are characteristic of postural hypotension, due to absence of baroreflex vasoconstrictor compensation for the venous pooling that occurs with upright tilting. Individuals without an active sympathetic nervous system also lack venoconstrictor nervous input to their venous system. In consequence, their veins are very compliant and this exaggerates venous pooling. Postural hypotension is most severe over the first few months after injury, probably because myogenic tone gradually develops in the vascular walls after this period, but it remains a long-term problem for many tetraplegic patients.

21.C. Since the underlying problem is excessive venous pooling under gravitational stress, mechanical compression of the dependent veins by use of elastic stockings and an abdominal binder minimizes postural hypotension. Avoiding rapid changes in posture is a second obvious approach, since this allows time for cerebrovascular autoregulation. In a minority of patients these strategies are not sufficient and ingestion of a vasoconstrictor substance such as ephedrine may be necessary.

Obviously, postural hypotension will be exaggerated by anything that causes peripheral vasodilation and so reduces total peripheral resistance. Patients therefore need to be counselled about the likely implications of rising soon after eating and of drinking alcohol. Restriction of water and sodium intakes will increase secretion of vasoconstrictor hormones but this does not help prevent postural hypotension, since there is simultaneous reduction of plasma volume.

22.C. Sean is fortunate that he has preservation of intact motor and sensory function at C_6. This allows wrist extension, arm movement and the use of some fingers, so he can type, reach out for light switches and perform a variety of motor tasks. However, he needs mechanical support for hand movements such as cleaning his teeth and using cutlery, because the motor pathways for wrist and finger flexion exit the spinal cord via C_7–C_8 nerves.

23.E. With a high spinal lesion, all of these aspects of reproductive function will be impaired. Erection is possible in some patients through activation of spinal reflexes or by use of penile implants. However, the reduced sperm count, reduced accessory gland secretions and retrograde ejaculation of semen into the bladder make it unlikely that intercourse will result in successful fertilization. Collection of semen for assisted conception is therefore the usual course of action.

24. A large proportion of individuals who suffer high spinal injury are young adults and the effect on their sexuality is a major concern to them and their partners. Because all sensory inputs from the genitalia to the brain travel via the spinal cord, orgasm is absent or at least very different from normal in high spinal patients of either gender. Unlike the situation in men, however, tetraplegia does not reduce fertility in women, since the events that contribute to early reproductive function do not rely on neural influences. Pregnancy progresses normally, although the physical presence of the pregnant uterus predisposes to pressure sores and urinary incontinence during the last few months. Perhaps surprisingly in view of the standard textbook view that oxytocin release relies on reflex signals from cervical mechanoreceptors, uterine contractions during parturition also develop normally. Nonetheless, there is no ability to contract abdominal muscles, so delivery may need to be assisted. As well, uterine contractions can initiate such severe sympathetic dysreflexia that there is dangerous elevation of blood pressure.

25. There is good long-term survival after low cervical lesions, provided that ventilatory function is maintained by assisted coughing and that there is effective monitoring for potentially dangerous respiratory and urinary tract infections. In patients with sufficient upper limb function, regular use of arm-strengthening exercises is valuable in maintaining mobility and manual control. But the absence of weight-bearing activities makes it difficult to avoid osteopenic changes in the skeleton and atrophy of lower limb muscles. Another common problem is chronic pain, usually but not always localized to dermatomes near the level of injury. The underlying mechanism is probably sprouting of damaged sensory neurons and formation of abnormal new connections, similar to the sequence of events that is thought to occur after injury to peripheral nerve trunks.

CASE REVIEW

Mechanical impact is likely to cause dislocation and spinal cord damage at levels of the spinal column that are most mobile. These are the lower cervical region, where the effects of hyperextension injury are most commonly seen, and T_8–T_{10}, which is the region most commonly affected by compression injury. About 50% of all these injuries result from motor vehicle accidents, with falls in the home (20%) and sporting accidents (15%) making up most of the rest. The current annual incidence is around 25 per million, so each year about 8000 people are admitted to spinal units in the USA and 1000 in the UK. Since in almost all cases the damage is permanent, it is easy to see that the total number of tetraplegic and paraplegic patients in the community is rising continually.

From the clinical viewpoint, cervical injury imposes by far the greater burden on patient and health care systems, because there is more serious immobilization and loss of independence than results from thoracic lesions. Even within the cervical region, however, the segmental level of injury has a major effect on outcome. Sean is fortunate that retention of intact spinal function above C_7 allows him to breathe spontaneously and to retain a reasonable degree of control of upper limb functions. This means that he can use a hand-driven wheelchair, carry out operations such as combing his hair, brushing his teeth and eating with minimal prosthetic support and can use his arms to help dress himself and assist in personal hygiene. If the lesion had occurred one segment higher up, then his motor control would have been substantially lessened by the loss of wrist extensor control. A lesion above the C_5 outflow would have removed all upper limb control, and one further segment rostrally would have inactivated his phrenic respiratory drive, necessitating a tracheostomy and mechanical ventilation.

Currently there is virtually no possibility of restoring normal neural functions below the level of a complete spinal lesion. The primary reason for this appears to be the physical barrier to axonal regrowth created by scar tissue at the injury site. However, there is in most cases relatively little neuronal death, so in theory regrowth could occur if the physical barrier was bypassed. Some experimental work has suggested that this might be achieved with implanted bridges containing neurotrophic chemicals, but any clinical application is still a long way off.

An alternative strategy is the implantation of electrodes, driven by computer programs that stimulate specific skeletal motor pathways. This might allow limb muscles to be activated in sequences that would allow locomotion, although of course there would be no restoration of sensory functions. Such prosthetic devices are likely to be commercially available within the lifespan of many current patients, emphasizing the practical value of maintaining their bone strength and muscle mass by physiotherapy.

KEY POINTS

- Traumatic cervical hyperextension is a common cause of spinal injury after motor and sporting accidents.
- If the level of spinal damage is above C_5, artificial ventilation is required but with lesions below this level spontaneous ventilation is preserved.
- With descending levels of damage over C_5–C_8 there is increasing preservation of upper limb function. Capacity to return to an independent lifestyle is critically dependent on the absolute segmental level of injury.

- Treatment of the tetraplegic patient must take into account both the absence of descending control pathways from brain to spinal cord and the fact that removal of this control allows reflex activation of spinal circuits below the level of injury.
- Some instances of these disinhibited reflexes, such as somatic muscle spasm, present a substantial clinical problem. Others afford potential benefits by giving the patient limited voluntary control over visceral functions.

ADDITIONAL READING

Bunge MB & Pearse DD (2003) Transplantation strategies to promote repair of the injured spinal cord. *Journal of Rehabilitation Research and Development* **40** (Suppl. 1): 55–62.

Glass CA (1999) *Spinal Cord Injury: Impact and Coping.* BPS Books, Leicester.

Grundy D & Swain A (2001) *ABC of Spinal Injury*, 4th edition. BMJ Publishing Group, London.

Sipski ML (2003) From the bench to the body: key issues associated with research aimed at a cure for SCI. *Journal of Rehabilitation Research and Development* **40** (Suppl. 1): 1–7.

Intermittent vomiting

CASE AND MCQS

Case introduction

Mrs J.L., aged 59, presents with a history of intermittent vomiting over the last 3 days. She has felt full and distended and she has vomited food that she ate 2–3 days earlier. Apart from the intermittent vomiting she feels reasonably well, and has continued to eat some food and drink fluids.

Her past history indicates that she has two children now aged 33 and 30, and there were no problems with her pregnancies. She was diagnosed with hypertension at the age of 54, and has been treated with a number of antihypertensive drugs. She is now on an angiotensin-converting enzyme (ACE) inhibitor and a low-dose diuretic in a combination tablet, and states that her blood pressure is well controlled at about 145/85 mmHg.

Mrs L. is thin; her weight is 61 kg (134 lb), height 1.70 m (5 ft, 7 in), blood pressure 125/75 mmHg, pulse rate 86 beats/min. Tissue turgor appears reduced. Her abdomen is not tender. There is a suggestion of fullness in the upper midline but no definite masses. No other abnormalities are found on examination.

She states that at the age of 48 she was diagnosed with duodenal ulcer for which she was treated with antacids and a histamine H_2-receptor antagonist (cimetidine). On a repeat gastroscopy it was stated that the ulcer was healed. She has had some indigestion since, but relatively infrequently. She takes an over-the-counter antacid intermittently, but usually has little indigestion.

Q1 Which of the following factors is the most potent direct stimulator of acid secretion?

A. gastrin
B. acetylcholine
C. vagal activity
D. histamine
E. alcohol

Q2 Which one of the following treatments is most effective to reduce or neutralize acid secretion and allow healing of a peptic ulcer?

A. sodium bicarbonate
B. inhibitors of vagal activity
C. a proton pump inhibitor
D. an H_1-antagonist
E. an H_2-antagonist

In questions 3 to 8 below, indicate which one of the below is the most appropriate response.

A number of hormones are produced by different structures located in the upper gastrointestinal tract. Some of the structures are:

A. fundus of the stomach
B. body of the stomach
C. antrum of the stomach
D. duodenum
E. pancreas

Q3 Which is the major site of gastrin production?

Q4 Which is the major site of gastric glands?

Q5 Which has the thickest musculature?

Q6 Which is the site of greatest muscle compliance?

Q7 Which is the major site of secretin production?

Q8 Which is the major site of cholecystokinin action?

Q9 In relation to the present episode, which of the following is the most likely cause of the vomiting?

A. food poisoning
B. small intestinal obstruction
C. large intestinal obstruction
D. pyloric obstruction
E. gastro-oesophageal sphincter obstruction

A diagnosis is made, and a nasogastric tube is passed and aspirated over the next 24 hours.

Q10 Once the distension and initial contents of the stomach have been removed, which of the options in Table 2.1 would be the most likely volume and composition of the 24-hour aspirate?

Table 2.1 Volume and composition options for Question 10

	Volume (ml/day)	pH	Sodium (mmol/l)	Potassium (mmol/l)	Chloride (mmol/l)
A	700	1.4	130	20	110
B	1100	2.5	50	14	120
C	1200	2.5	50	14	60
D	1200	3	130	14	120
E	2500	3	50	30	60

Consider the likely effects on plasma composition and plasma volume of vomiting gastric contents for several days followed by gastric aspiration for 24 hours, assuming that there was no fluid replacement given.

Typical normal values for plasma composition are as follows:

Osmolality	290 mosmol/l
pH	7.40
Sodium	140 mmol/l
Potassium	4.0 mmol/l
Chloride	92 mmol/l
Bicarbonate	25 mmol/l

Table 2.2 Plasma profiles for Question 11

	Osmolality (mmol/l)	pH	Sodium (mmol/l)	Potassium (mmol/l)	Chloride (mmol/l)	Bicarbonate (mmol/l)
A	270	7.48	130	3.1	87	38
B	290	7.35	145	4.0	100	28
C	290	7.48	130	3.1	87	38
D	295	7.48	148	4.0	87	30
E	295	7.48	148	3.1	87	38

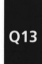

Q11 Which of the profiles shown in Table 2.2 is the most likely plasma profile after vomiting and gastric aspiration?

At the end of 24 hours, the following values (see below) were found for Mrs L., related to the 24-hour gastric aspirate and for the plasma electrolytes.

These data indicate that she was slightly dehydrated (high plasma sodium) and had a hypokalaemic alkalosis. In addition, she has poor tissue turgor and low blood pressure, suggesting volume depletion.

Gastric juice:

Volume	1200 ml/day
pH	2.3
Sodium	50 mmol/l
Potassium	12 mmol/l
Chloride	110 mmol/l

Plasma:

Osmolality	295 mosmol/l
pH	7.48
Sodium	147 mmol/l
Potassium	3.1 mmol/l
Chloride	86 mmol/l
Bicarbonate	35 mmol/l

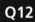

Q12 What is the cause of her low plasma potassium?

A. removal of potassium in the gastric aspirate
B. excessive loss of potassium in the urine
C. movement of potassium into cells
D. A, B and C
E. A and B

Q13 A urine collection was done over a 4-hour period during this time. How would the results compare with that expected in a normal individual? Select which of the options in Table 2.3 you think is the most likely result.

Table 2.3 Options for Question 13

	Volume	pH	NH$_4^+$	Sodium
A	0	↑	0	0
B	↓	↑	↓	↓
C	↓	↓	0	↓
D	↑	↓	↑	0
E	↑	0	↑	↑

(↑ = an increase from normal, ↓ = a decrease from normal, 0 = no variation from normal).

Q14 As stated above, Mrs L. has alkalosis. Her body will attempt to correct this by altering urine excretion, but there will also be acute alterations in respiratory function so as to blunt the change in pH. Which of the following is the most likely to occur?

A. intermittent breathing
B. shallow, rapid breathing
C. deep rapid breathing
D. deep slow breathing
E. slow shallow breathing

Table 2.4 A selection of abnormal acid–base values for arterial plasma

	pH	P_{CO_2}, mmHg (kPa)	Bicarbonate (mmol/l)	P_{O_2}, mmHg (kPa)
A	7.48	50 (6.7)	22	100 (13.3)
B	7.44	48 (6.4)	30	95 (12.7)
C	7.44	30 (4.0)	19	95 (12.7)
D	7.35	30 (4.0)	19	95 (12.7)
E	7.32	50 (4.0)	33	80 (10.7)

Typical normal acid–base values for arterial plasma are:

pH	7.35–7.45
P_{CO_2}	35–45 mmHg (4.6–6.0 kPa)
Bicarbonate	22–28 mmol/l
P_{O_2}	85–95 mmHg (11.3–12.7 kPa)

Table 2.4 (above) lists a selection of abnormal data for these parameters.

Q15 Which set of values in Table 2.4 is most compatible with metabolic alkalosis?

Q16 Which set of values in Table 2.4 is most compatible with respiratory alkalosis?

Q17 Which set of values in Table 2.4 is most compatible with metabolic acidosis?

Table 2.5 shows a number of different urine compositions, indicating the change in some electrolyte concentrations from their usual values .

Table 2.5 A selection of different urine compositions

	Sodium	Potassium	Bicarbonate	NH_4^+
A	↑	↑	↑	↓
B	↓	↑	↑	↓
C	0	0 or ↓	↓	↑
D	↑	↑	↑	0
E	0	0 or ↑	↑	↓

(↑ = an increase from normal, ↓ = a decrease from normal, 0 = no variation from normal)

Q18 Which composition in Table 2.5 is most compatible with metabolic alkalosis due to repeated vomiting or gastric aspiration?

Q19 Which composition in Table 2.5 is most compatible with metabolic acidosis due to a drug that inhibits secretion of hydrogen ions by the proximal tubule of the kidney?

Q20 Which composition in Table 2.5 is most compatible with metabolic alkalosis due to sodium bicarbonate ingestion?

Q21 Which composition in Table 2.5 is most compatible with respiratory alkalosis?

Q22 Which composition in Table 2.5 is most compatible with respiratory acidosis?

Q23 Which of the following procedures would be most useful to correct Mrs L.'s metabolic alkalosis?

A. volume expansion with infusion of normal saline
B. ammonium chloride administration
C. a carbonic anhydrase inhibitor
D. sodium bicarbonate infusion
E. none of the above

Q24 Which of the following would be the most useful fluid replacement to give her over the next 24 hours?

A. 3 litres of normal saline + potassium supplementation
B. 1 litre of normal saline + 1 litre of 5% glucose in distilled water + potassium supplementation
C. 3 litres of normal saline
D. 3 litres of normal saline + 1 litre of 5% glucose in distilled water + potassium supplementation
E. 1 litre of normal saline + sodium bicarbonate + potassium supplementation

Over the next 24 hours, Mrs L. was given fluids as decided in the last question. Her plasma chemistry at the end of this time showed:

Sodium	144 mmol/l
Potassium	3.8 mmol/l
Bicarbonate	31 mmol/l
pH	7.44
P_{CO_2}	48 mmHg (6.4 kPa)

Her urine output increased and the amounts of sodium and bicarbonate in the urine rose.

Investigations revealed an obstruction at the pylorus. Three days after admission and after decompression of her stomach and correction of the volume and electrolyte disturbances, surgery was undertaken to bypass the obstruction.

Mrs L. made a good recovery.

MCQ ANSWERS AND FEEDBACK

1.D. All of these can stimulate acid secretion by the oxyntic (parietal) cells of the gastric gland. Gastrin is a potent stimulant that works indirectly by releasing histamine from the endocrine cell of the gastric gland. Acetylcholine, released by vagal activity, stimulates acid secretion directly by the oxyntic cell. Vagal activity also causes gastrin release. Alcohol increases acid secretion. Histamine, however, is the most potent direct stimulator of acid secretion.

2.C. H_1-antagonists have no effect on acid secretion, which is however reduced by H_2-antagonists. Sodium bicarbonate neutralizes acid, but total acid secretion is increased due to inhibition of the usual feedback. Inhibition of vagal activity reduces acid secretion, but the most effective way is directly to inhibit the proton pump K^+/H^+ ATPase on the luminal membrane.

3.C. Gastrin is produced by gastrin (G) cells in the antrum. There is also some produced by G cells in the duodenum. The delta cell of the pancreas produces somatostatin, but has the potential to produce gastrin when a tumour of this cell occurs (Zollinger–Ellison syndrome).

4.B. The gastric glands that secrete acid, pepsinogen and intrinsic factor are predominantly in the body of the stomach.

5.C. The muscle in the walls of gastric antrum and pylorus is much thicker than that in other parts of the stomach or in the intestine.

6.A. The fundus of the stomach is easily distended (i.e. has the greatest compliance), allowing large meals to be eaten with little discomfort.

7.D. Secretin is produced by cells in the duodenal mucosa, and it is released when acid is in the duodenum. Secretin acts on the pancreatic duct cells to cause bicarbonate secretion.

8.E. Cholecystokinin released from cells in the duodenum acts on the gallbladder to cause contraction, and also on pancreatic acinus cells to cause enzyme secretion. It does act also on the stomach to inhibit the action of gastrin, but its major actions are on gallbladder and pancreas.

9.D. The episode is not suggestive of acute food poisoning and with acute large or small bowel obstruction she would be much sicker. Obstruction at the gastro-oesophageal sphincter would be likely to be associated with more chronic pain and with vomiting immediately after food.

10.B. The sodium concentration in A and D is too high, and the chloride in C and E is too low, so the most likely answer is B. Note that this causes loss of water in excess of the plasma concentration of electrolytes, leading to dehydration as well as volume depletion.

11.E. The loss of H^+ would tend to increase pH, that is, cause alkalosis. Thus B is incorrect. The loss of water in excess of sodium would tend to cause high plasma sodium. Thus A and C are incorrect. Potassium would tend to fall due to its urinary loss and also due to the alkalosis causing cellular uptake of potassium. Thus B and D are unlikely. E is the most likely, and this is supported by the low chloride and high bicarbonate.

12.D. Potassium is lost in the gastric aspirate. The alkalosis moves potassium into cells, and the loss of bicarbonate in the urine will cause a high potential difference in the collecting tubules and duct, producing greater potassium secretion and loss in the urine.

13.B. The urine volume would be down due to plasma volume depletion. Thus the correct answer is B or C. The pH would be increased due to the alkalosis and high bicarbonate in plasma – that is, statement B. Because the pH is increased, urine ammonium is reduced. Sodium excretion is down despite the high plasma sodium because of the volume depletion.

14.E. There is an alkalosis and high plasma bicarbonate. The Henderson–Hasselbalch equation (pH = 6.1 + log [bicarbonate]/$0.03.P_{CO_2}$ in mmHg) shows that pH stability requires the ratio of [bicarbonate] to $0.03.P_{CO_2}$ to be kept close to 20. As bicarbonate has risen, P_{CO_2} will also have to be elevated. This is achieved by slow, shallow breathing, which retains CO_2 in the blood.

15.B. In metabolic alkalosis, the pH rises but may not be outside the normal range. Bicarbonate will be elevated, and there will be a compensatory increase in P_{CO_2}. Only answer B meets these conditions. The ratio of [bicarbonate]/$0.03.P_{CO_2}$ will stay close to 20:1.

16.C. Respiratory alkalosis occurs due to hyperventilation blowing off CO_2. Thus P_{CO_2} will be reduced – that is, C or D. Bicarbonate will also fall due to metabolic compensation – that is, C or D). However the pH in C is on the high side of normal, while in D it is on the low side of normal. Thus C is the correct answer.

17.D. In metabolic acidosis, protons are retained. These react with bicarbonate to cause a fall in plasma bicarbonate (C or D). The P_{CO_2} will also fall due to respiratory compensation (C or D). The pH in D is less than the pH in C, and is on the acidic side of normal. Thus D is the correct answer.

18.B. In metabolic alkalosis, there would be increased bicarbonate and potassium and also increased or unaltered sodium in the urine. However, with volume depletion as would exist under these circumstances, the urine sodium would be down (see Question 13). Bicarbonate would be increased usually but, if volume depletion is severe, it may all be reabsorbed in the proximal tubule, preventing its excretion in the urine. This urinary loss of bicarbonate is what corrects the alkalosis.

19.A. In metabolic acidosis, the pH of blood and of urine would usually move in the same direction, leading to a low urine bicarbonate and increased urine ammonium. However, if H^+ secretion is inhibited, this means that bicarbonate is not all reabsorbed. Thus urinary bicarbonate increases, pH rises, and there is less ammonium. There will also be increased sodium as H^+ secretion is involved in sodium re-absorption. Potassium excretion will be increased due to a higher potential difference in the collecting tubule and duct, resulting from a higher concentration of bicarbonate at this site.

20.A. Sodium and bicarbonate are both increased due to the extra filtered load (see Question 18). Potassium secretion in the distal nephron is increased, due to more bicarbonate causing a high potential difference. Ammonium concentration is down, as H^+ secreted in the distal nephron is used to reabsorb bicarbonate.

21.E. In respiratory alkalosis, the Pa_{CO_2} is low. Thus bicarbonate must be lost in order to maintain the ratio of [bicarbonate]/$0.03.P_{CO_2}$ close to 20:1. The loss of bicarbonate in the urine means that the urine has a high pH, thus ammonium is low. There should be little effect on sodium excretion. Potassium would tend to rise due to the high level of bicarbonate in the distal nephron.

22.C. In respiratory acidosis, H^+ is elevated and Pa_{CO_2} is high. H^+ ions are secreted in the tubule fluid, and this causes reabsorption of all the bicarbonate. The H^+ then combines with NH_3 to form ammonium. There should be little effect on sodium excretion. Potassium excretion would be little affected.

23.A. Metabolic alkalosis is self-correcting unless there is volume depletion, as the high plasma bicarbonate exceeds the renal threshold and bicarbonate is lost in the urine. Thus, in order to correct alkalosis it is essential to expand plasma volume.

24.D. The patient needs replacement of her continuing losses and of the deficit that already exists. Thus at least 3–4 litres of fluid are needed in the next 24 hours, and maybe even more. It should not all be saline, as there is some dehydration present – that is, water has been lost in excess of electrolytes due to the vomiting and the gastric aspirate. Potassium has also been lost and some potassium supplementation is required; typically around 30 mmol. Answer D satisfies these requirements best.

CASE REVIEW

This patient presented with a previous history of an ulcer that had been treated with cimetidine (an H_2-receptor antagonist) and she stated that the ulcer had healed. However, she subsequently had indigestion which she treated with over-the-counter medication, suggesting that there was still ulcer activity proceeding.

It is now known that the cause of a large number of ulcers is the organism *Helicobacter pylori*. Excessive secretion of acid is an important mechanistic step leading to ulcer formation. Neutralization of acid or prevention of acid secretion leads to healing of the ulcer but not to a cure, and recurrence is frequent when medication is stopped.

Hydrochloric acid is secreted by the parietal (oxyntic) cell of the gastric gland by an H^+/K^+ ATPase proton pump (Fig. 2.1).

	produces	
Parietal (oxyntic) cell	→	HCl
	→	B_{12}/ intrinsic factor
Peptic cell	→	Pepsinogen
Endocrine (ECL) cell	→	Histamine
Mucous cell	→	Mucus

Fig. 2.1 Secretions of the gastric glands

This secretion is directly stimulated by histamine, binding to the adenyl cyclase receptor complex and increasing cellular cyclic AMP. It is also stimulated by acetylcholine, working via cytosolic calcium. Histamine binds to an H_2-type receptor and blocking this receptor reduces acid secretion. The most effective blockade, however, is by inhibiting the proton pump. Gastrin is produced in G cells located in the antrum at the stomach and acts on the endocrine enterochromaffin-like (ECL) cells of the gastric gland, located in the body of the stomach. These cells release histamine, which stimulates local acid secretion (Fig. 2.2). Gastrin also acts on stomach muscles, increasing the rate and force of contraction, and has a trophic effect that improves the growth of many cells of the gastro-intestinal tract.

This patient's ulcer was located in the pyloric region of the stomach. Its intermittent recurrence and healing had eventually led to pyloric obstruction by accumulated fibrous scar tissue. The initial treatment of pyloric obstruction is to relieve stomach distension via a nasogastric tube and then later to relieve the obstruction by surgery.

The normal amount of gastric juice secreted is between 1000 and 2000 ml/day. The chloride concentration is close to or above that of plasma and the anionic component is made up of sodium, potassium and H^+. The pH is below 3.0 and at the gastric gland it would be close to 1.0. Thus aspiration of gastric juice will lead to loss of water, sodium, potassium, H^+ and chloride. The loss of water is in excess of electrolytes (that is, compared with plasma composition) and thus the patient would tend to become dehydrated, with a rise in plasma osmolality as well as being volume depleted.

The loss of chloride means that plasma chloride will fall, bicarbonate will rise (due to loss of H^+ ions) and pH will rise; that is, loss of H^+ ions leads to a lower plasma H^+ ion concentration. Potassium will fall due to gastric loss of potassium and to cellular uptake of potassium caused by the alkalosis. Sodium is lost from the body but the loss of water is in excess and thus plasma osmolality and sodium concentration both rise.

To correct the volume depletion the kidney retains fluid, so urinary volume falls. Urine pH will be above 7.4 due to bicarbonate excretion. There will be no ammonium (as no H^+ ions are available) and urinary sodium will be low even though plasma

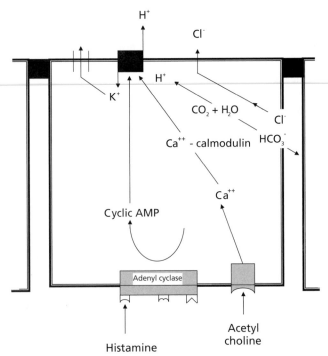

Fig. 2.2 Histamine released from the ECL (endocrine cell) of the gastric gland in response to gastrin and acetylcholine (vagal activity) binds to a receptor linked to the stimulatory subunit of the adenyl cyclase to increase cyclic AMP production. This increases activity of the H^+–potassium (proton) pump. Acetylcholine causes entry of Ca^{2+} which releases Ca^{2+} from the endoplasmic reticulum. This calcium links to calmodulin and increases the proton pump activity. Adenyl cyclase activity can be reduced by substances (somatostatin, opioid, prostanoids, etc.) binding to receptors linked to the inhibitory subunit of adenyl cyclase.

sodium is high. The retention of sodium is a mechanism to retain water and to correct the volume depletion and the stimulus for aldosterone secretion is not usually the sodium concentration. Provided a patient is adequately volume expanded the alkalosis will self-correct due to loss of bicarbonate in the urine. However if there is volume depletion there will be excessive absorption of bicarbonate in the proximal tubule (Fig. 2.3).

There will also be alterations in respiratory function. To maintain pH close to the normal value the CO_2 in plasma must rise (to balance a high bicarbonate) and thus there will be slow, shallow breathing. Blood gases will show a pH at the upper end or above the normal range, bicarbonate and P_{CO_2} above the normal range, and oxygen in the normal range.

To correct the volume depletion and alkalosis, Mrs L. was given normal saline. In addition, glucose in distilled water was needed to correct the dehydration. Also, potassium needed to be provided to correct the hypokalaemia. A surgical procedure was required to relieve the obstruction, and assessment would need to be made post-operatively of whether a curative procedure to treat *Helicobacter pylori* must be undertaken.

$$pH = pK + \log \frac{A^-}{HA} \qquad \text{(for any buffer)}$$

$$pH = 6.1 + \log \frac{HCO_3^-}{H_2CO_3} \qquad (H_2CO_3 \bullet HCO_3^- + H^+)$$

$$= 6.1 + \log \frac{HCO_3^-}{(0.03\ pCO_2)} \qquad \text{(parameter measured is } CO_2\text{)}$$

$$pH = 6.1 + \log \frac{24}{(0.03)\ 40} \qquad \text{(usual values)}$$

$$= 6.1 + \log 20 \qquad \text{(ratio of } HCO_3^- : 0.03\ PCO_2 \text{ usually about 20)}$$

$$= 7.4 \qquad \text{(usual pH)}$$

Fig. 2.3 The Henderson–Hasselbalch equation. Note that the pH is protected. Thus, if bicarbonate levels fall (metabolic acidosis) pH would fall, but $P\text{co}_2$ falls due to hyperventilation and pH change is minimized. If $P\text{co}_2$ rises (e.g. respiratory insufficiency) the pH would fall. The change is minimized by a rise in plasma HCO_3^- with less excretion by the kidney and the pH change is minimized.

KEY POINTS

- Excess secretion of acid is important in the formation of gastric ulcers.
- Infection with *Helicobacter pylori* is an important cause of gastric ulceration.
- The gastric glands secrete HCl, pepsinogen, intrinsic factor and mucus.
- Pepsinogen is activated by a low pH.
- Vagal activity, acetylcholine, gastrin and histamine directly or indirectly stimulate acid secretion.

- Loss of gastric juice leads to a hypokalaemic alkalosis with volume depletion and dehydration.
- Respiratory compensation attempts to correct the alkalosis by slow respiration elevating the CO_2 content of plasma.
- Provided there is no volume depletion, the kidney corrects alkalosis by the loss of HCO_3^- in the urine.

ADDITIONAL READING

Beales IL (2004) The management of peptic ulcer disease. *Practitioner* **248**: 524–9.

Braunwald E, Fauci AS, Kasper DL *et al.* (2001) *Harrison's Principles of Internal Medicine*, 15th edition. McGraw-Hill, New York.

Johnson LR (2001) *Gastrointestinal Physiology*, 6th edition. Mosby, St. Louis.

Rose BD & Post TW (2001) *Clinical Physiology of Acid Base and Electrolyte Disorders*, 5th edition. McGraw-Hill, New York.

Seldin DW & Giebisch G (2000) *The Kidney: Physiology and Pathophysiology*, 3rd edition. Lippincott Williams & Wilkins, Philadelphia.

High pressure at sea

CASES AND MCQS

Case introduction

You are a practitioner with an interest in respiratory medicine and apply for a three-month appointment as medical superintendent on a diving expedition to research wrecks in a remote area of the Indian Ocean.

In addition to general medical care of the crew and diving team, your duties will include drawing up guidelines for the diving schedule, supervision of apparatus and air supplies, and ongoing assessment of the divers for any complications of their work.

As a background to thinking about the particulars of hyperbaric physiology and medicine, it is helpful to start by remembering some basics of respiratory function.

 Q1 During a maximal inspiratory effort, intrapleural and intrapulmonary pressures would be expected to reach peak values (relative to atmospheric) of around:

A. intrapleural −5 mmHg (−0.7 kPa), intrapulmonary −2 mmHg (−0.3 kPa)
B. intrapleural −5 mmHg (−0.7 kPa), intrapulmonary +5 mmHg (0.3 kPa)
C. intrapleural +82 mmHg (11 kPa), intrapulmonary +90 mmHg (12 kPa)
D. intrapleural −82 mmHg (−11 kPa), intrapulmonary −90 mmHg (−12 kPa)
E. intrapleural −82 mmHg (−11 kPa), intrapulmonary −75 mmHg (−10 kPa)

Q2 If an individual swimming underwater were to breathe through a hose open to the air above water level, the maximum depth at which this person could stay submerged would be less than 1 m (3 ft). The factor that determines this limit is:

A. reduced alveolar Po_2 because the lung is compressed by external pressure
B. reduced alveolar Po_2 due to the extra anatomical dead space of the hose
C. inability of respiratory muscles to overcome external thoracic compression
D. inability of respiratory muscles to overcome the extra resistance of the hose
E. inability of respiratory muscles to overcome the increased density of air at high pressure

Before going on, let us revise the relationship between inspired oxygen concentration and oxygen delivery. You will recall that, normally, alveolar Po_2 (PAo_2) is around 50 mmHg (6.5 kPa) lower than atmospheric Po_2 because the inspired air is diluted with water vapour and carbon dioxide. There is also a further fall in Po_2 between alveolar air, where it is typically 100 mmHg (13 kPa), and systemic arterial plasma, where it is typically about 5 mmHg (0.7 kPa) lower.

Q3 | The arterial P_{O_2} (P_{aO_2}) is normally lower than that in the alveolar air because:

A. blood transits the pulmonary capillaries too quickly for equilibration of oxygen between air and plasma
B. not all of the left cardiac output has passed through the pulmonary circulation
C. not all of the pulmonary blood flow is exposed to alveolar air
D. both B and C
E. all of A, B and C

Q4 | If the composition of inspired air altered so that P_{AO_2} was reduced from 100 mmHg to 80 mmHg (from 13 to 10.7 kPa) and P_{aO_2} was reduced from 95 mmHg to 75 mmHg (from 12.7 to 10 kPa), what would be the consequence for oxygen carriage?

A fall in P_{aO_2} from 95 mmHg (12.7 kPa) to 75 mmHg (10 kPa) would correspond to arterial blood carrying:
A. the same amount of oxygen as before
B. 5% less oxygen than before
C. 20% less oxygen than before
D. 50% less oxygen than before
E. 75% less oxygen than before

Let us now turn to assessment of the individuals who have volunteered to act as divers on this expedition. Evaluating their suitability will first involve assessing their physical fitness.

Q5 | The standard parameter used for evaluating physical fitness is the subject's $V_{O_{2max}}$ – the amount of oxygen consumed per unit time at maximal workload. A fit, 20-year-old man would be expected to have a $V_{O_{2max}}$ around:

A. 10 (ml/min)/kg
B. 20 (ml/min)/kg
C. 40 (ml/min)/kg
D. 60 (ml/min)/kg
E. 80 (ml/min)/kg

Next, you need to exclude any factors that might interfere with survival in an environment that involves high pressures and a limited source of gas exchange. J.P., one of the volunteers you examine (38 years, BMI 28, height 184 cm (6 ft)), shows the following results (right) of standard lung function tests:

Forced vital capacity	4200 ml
FEV$_1$	3400 ml
Inspiratory capacity (measured by spirometry)	2800 ml
Functional residual capacity (measured by helium dilution)	2200 ml
Peak inspiratory flow rate	6.0 litres/s
Peak expiratory flow rate (measured by peak flow meter)	8.4 litres/s

Q6 | Calculate J.P.'s total lung capacity (TLC) and residual volume (RV):

A. TLC 6400 ml, RV 1200 ml
B. TLC 5400 ml, RV 1200 ml
C. TLC 4200 ml, RV 2200 ml
D. TLC 5000 ml, RV 800 ml
E. TLC 4200 ml, RV 800 ml

Q7 | On the basis of these findings, J.P. appears to have:

A. normal lung function
B. restrictive lung disease due to intrapulmonary factors
C. restrictive lung disease due to muscular insufficiency
D. obstructive lung disease due to intrapulmonary factors
E. obstructive lung disease due to tracheal stenosis

The largest group of prospective divers who require careful respiratory assessment are people with asthma. It has been suggested that the uneven ventilation that occurs in many asthmatic lungs could result in air trapping, with lung rupture and potential air embolism during ascent from a dive. Some practitioners, however, maintain that there is little or no epidemiological evidence for this occurring.

There is, on the other hand, universal agreement that asthmatic individuals are highly susceptible to attacks of exercise-induced asthma during scuba use. Because of this, asthma is generally viewed as a contraindication to employment as a commercial diver. Interestingly, swimming itself has been shown to be less likely than running to provoke exercise-induced asthma.

Q8 Why should scuba diving tend to precipitate exercise-induced asthma when swimming itself does not?

Assessment of hearing and vestibular function is another essential aspect of screening prospective divers and damage to these functions is the most common area of medical problems associated with diving.

Remember that the inner ear is open to the cerebrospinal fluid, so inner ear pressure changes in parallel with atmospheric pressure, but that equilibration of middle ear and atmospheric pressures relies on the Eustachian tube (auditory tube). This equilibration is vital since rupture of the tympanic membrane can occur with pressure differentials as low as 100 mmHg (13 kPa).

The nasopharyngeal ostium of the tube is usually kept closed by tissue pressure and opens only if middle ear pressure rises or if the tissues around the ostium are mobilized, for example by swallowing. However, if middle ear pressure falls more than 90 mmHg (12 kPa) below atmospheric then the ostium is sucked shut and cannot usually be opened even by vigorous swallowing (Fig. 3.1).

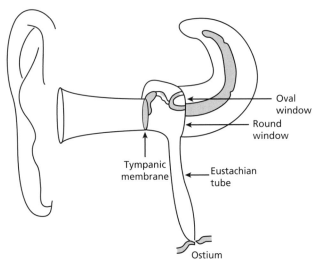

Fig. 3.1 Relationship of the three ear chambers and the Eustachian tube.

With this background information, think about the potential problems of middle ear stability during changes in atmospheric pressure.

Q9 Will middle ear pressure stability be harder to ensure during descent or ascent, and why? During descent, at what absolute depth will it become impossible to perform pressure equilibration and at what depth might eardrum rupture occur in the absence of this equilibration?

Damage to the tympanic membrane is characteristically associated with severe pain and also, if water enters the middle ear, with sensations of dizziness. In addition, vomiting can occur because of damage to the membrane's nerve supply.

Q10 The sensory nerve supply to the tympanic membrane is from:

A. cranial V, VI and VIII
B. cranial V, VII and VIII
C. cranial V, VII and IX
D. cranial V, VIII and IX
E. cranial V, IX and X

Because of the continual danger of ear damage, it is essential that prospective divers have accurate baseline measurements of auditory capacity and that their hearing is monitored regularly during a dive trip. Under field conditions, sophisticated audiometric testing is not usually practicable, so it is necessary to be familiar with the standard hearing tests that use a tuning fork.

The main purpose of these tests is to determine whether any hearing loss is due to damage to the middle ear (that is, *conduction* damage) or to the inner ear (*neurosensory* damage). Distinguishing between these may not be obvious from other signs of injury but is often essential for appropriate clinical handling.

Rinne's test involves comparing the sound heard when it is transmitted to the ear normally through air with that heard after conduction through the skull. The patient is asked whether the sound of a tuning fork is louder and lasts longer when the fork is placed against the tip of the mastoid bone or when it is held about 5 cm outside the ear canal.

Think about the logic of sound movement through the components of the ear and answer this question.

Q11 With Rinne's test, a patient with inner ear deafness will report that:

A. the sound is louder and longer with air conduction
B. the sound is louder and longer with bone conduction
C. the sound is louder but shorter with air conduction
D. the sound is louder but shorter with bone conduction
E. both air and bone conduction give similar results

Weber's test is applied to situations where only one ear is affected. It relies on the fact that perception of specific sounds is normally limited by the continual background noise that impinges on the middle ear amplifier. The test involves placing a tuning fork on the midline of the patient's skull, usually on the forehead or the vortex pilorum.

Q12 With Weber's test, a patient with unilateral middle ear deafness will report that:

A. the sound is louder in the normal ear
B. the sound is louder in the affected ear
C. the sound is not heard in the affected ear
D. the sound is heard for longer in the normal ear
E. the sound is similar in both ears

The most widely publicized problem with diving is decompression sickness (also known as 'the bends' and 'caisson disease'). This is caused by the formation of bubbles of nitrogen within tissues and the bloodstream during reduction of ambient pressure after a period of hyperbaric exposure.

The time that a diver can stay submerged without the need for decompression falls very rapidly with increasing depth (Fig. 3.2).

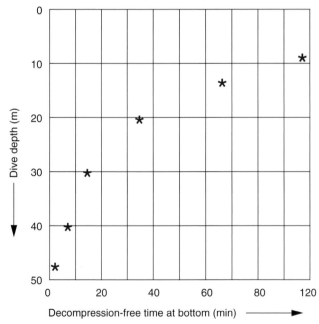

Fig. 3.2 Duration of dives that can be undertaken safely without staged decompression at different dive depths. Note that the times shown are for the purposes of illustration and should not be used for actual diving.

Rapid ascent is possible after staying at 8 m (27 ft) for over 3 hours but descending only another 3 m (10 ft) reduces this safe time to less than 2 hours and at 40 m (130 ft) depth it is only 8 minutes. With longer periods of submersion, the diver needs to spend time equilibrating during the ascent process. The time needed for adequate decompression is, as with the decompression-free time, extremely dependent on dive depth (Fig. 3.3).

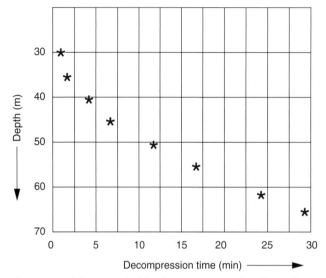

Fig. 3.3 Total times needed for decompression after dives of 15 minutes duration to various depths. Note that the times shown are for the purposes of illustration and should not be used for actual diving.

Because the inspired air that equilibrates with body fluids contains large amounts of both oxygen and nitrogen, we should be clear on why the need for decompression is related specifically to nitrogen.

Q13 The need for decompression during ascent is due specifically to the behaviour of nitrogen in the body because:

A. inspired air contains much more nitrogen than oxygen
B. nitrogen is less water-soluble than oxygen
C. nitrogen is more water-soluble than oxygen
D. at sea level, the body fluids contain more dissolved nitrogen than oxygen
E. nitrogen is an inert gas

The present expedition is concerned with a wreck that is lodged on a relatively shallow reef (depth 5–10 m, 17–33 ft) but the contents of which have spilled over the reef's edge and are estimated to be lying at around 60 m (190 ft).

One of your responsibilities will be to liaise with the diving master on the gas mixtures required by the salvage team. The ship's dive shop has capacity to produce both compressed air and a range of combinations of oxygen with nitrogen and helium. Look at the sample mixtures listed below and consider which would be suitable for specific uses.

A. 100% oxygen
B. 50% oxygen, 50% nitrogen
C. 50% oxygen, 50% helium
D. 21% oxygen, 79% nitrogen
E. 21% oxygen, 79% helium
F. 10% oxygen, 90% nitrogen
G. 10% oxygen, 90% helium
H. 3% oxygen, 97% nitrogen
I. 3% oxygen, 97% helium

Q14 Which of the above would be the best choice for use by a diver working for periods of 2–3 hours at a depth of 6 m (20 ft)?

Q15 Which of the above would be the best choice for use by a diver who has to descend for 5–10 minutes to a depth of 60 m (190 ft)?

Q16 Which of the above would be the best choice for use by a diver working for periods of 1–2 hours at a depth of 60 m (190 ft)?

With professional crews, diving accidents are now relatively uncommon because the underlying problems associated with hyperbaric exposure are well understood. On this expedition, you encounter only two significant mishaps, both of which coincidently occur within a day of each other.

The first of these takes place during work on the main wreck site at a depth of 10 m (33 ft). One of the divers, who has been loading artefacts into a hoist for about 20 minutes, cuts his hand deeply. He ascends rapidly, keeping his glottis open during ascent.

Q17 If the diver's end-inspiratory lung volume was 3 litres at a depth of 10 m (33 ft) and he had held his breath during ascent, what would his lung volume be at sea level?

A. 1.5 litres
B. 3 litres
C. 4.5 litres
D. 6 litres
E. 12 litres

As he climbs onto the deck, he complains of a sharp pain under his left arm that started during ascent and he says that he now feels breathless. On examination, you see that respiratory movements of the chest wall are slightly smaller on his left than his right side. Chest sounds are normal and there is no irregularity of heart rate or blood pressure. During examination, he spits up approximately 20 ml of bright red blood.

The ship has no imaging facilities for confirmation but from the symptomology you suspect that he has a small, simple left-side pneumothorax. Although divers are trained to keep an open glottis during ascent, air sometimes becomes trapped in a lung lobule, rupturing the parenchyma and potentially tearing the overlying pleura.

Q18 The risk of air trapping in the lung during ascent would be increased under the circumstances described for this diver because of:

A. airway constriction due to hyperoxia
B. airway constriction due to hypercapnia
C. dehydration of the airways mucosa by dry inspired air
D. increased density of inspired air at depth
E. head-down position during working at depth

The patient is given analgesics to reduce his pleuritic pain and 100% oxygen for his breathlessness. The absence of pronounced reduction in chest wall excursion or of a mediosternal shift indicates that his pneumothorax is small in size. In these circumstances it is not useful to aspirate air from the pleural space: it will be absorbed spontaneously over several weeks. Continued oxygen treatment is unnecessary and the patient should be encouraged to be normally active, but without vigorous exercise, until the lesion has healed fully. Radiographic verification of healing would be reassuring.

The second incident occurs during hoisting of salvaged materials, when a cable jams and one of the divers has to go down to free it. The dive depth is an estimated 60 m (190 ft) but the bottom time is not expected to be more than 5 minutes, so there is no need for a special gas mixture. The diver takes a full cylinder and descends rapidly, using weights. It takes only 3 minutes to free the cable and he then resurfaces and climbs on deck, but collapses immediately. He is semi-conscious and complains of dizziness, nausea and a severe headache, which he says were not present before he ascended. His skin colour is normal.

You start to administer 100% oxygen via a facemask and measure his haemoglobin saturation using a pulse oximeter on his ear lobe. This indicates a saturation of approximately 70%. He is taken to the ship's hyperbaric chamber and ventilated with oxygen at 2 atm (202 kPa) pressure for 3 hours. At the end of this time, his haemoglobin saturation is 88% and his symptoms are minimal.

Analysis of the air in the cylinder that was used for the dive shows the following:

Q19 What values would be expected for normal air?

Investigation reveals that the normal compressor used for filling air cylinders was serviced during the day and that a back-up compressor had been used to fill the last cylinder. Inspection of this compressor shows a fault in the exhaust system, so that small amounts of exhaust can be sucked into the main air intake under some circumstances.

The symptoms shown by the diver, his reduced haemoglobin saturation and the rapid response to ventilation with oxygen are all consistent with carbon monoxide poisoning. However, there appears to be a mismatch between the amount of carbon monoxide present and the effect on haemoglobin. Carbon monoxide binds to the oxygen-binding site of haemoglobin 250 times as effectively as oxygen itself. But look at the CO/haemoglobin dissociation curve shown in Fig. 3.4. You can see that a P_{CO} of 0.015 mmHg (0.002 kPa) is not high enough to cause any haemoglobin inactivation, whereas we know from the oximeter reading that in fact only 70% of the haemoglobin binding sites could carry oxygen.

There is also the paradox that the diver was clearly in a state of severe hypoxia although 70% saturation of haemoglobin with oxygen would still allow his arterial blood to carry 14 ml oxygen/100 ml, a considerably higher amount than the resting oxygen consumption of around 5 ml/100 ml.

Finally, it is puzzling that although he was breathing from the contaminated cylinder throughout the dive, he did not exhibit symptoms of poisoning until he surfaced.

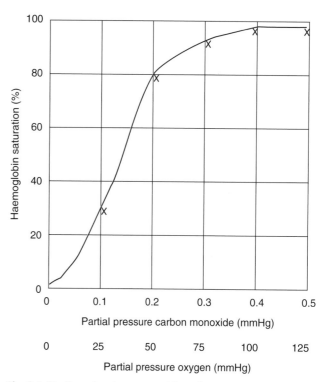

Fig. 3.4 Binding of carbon monoxide and oxygen to haemoglobin. Note that the shape of the dissociation curve is identical to that for both gases except for the fact that the concentration of carbon monoxide needed to achieve any particular level of saturation is 250 times lower.

Q20 What explanation can you give for the disparities between carbon monoxide concentration, the percentage inactivation of haemoglobin and the apparent degree of hypoxia? And why did the effects of poisoning appear only when the diver surfaced rather than when he was at depth?

Effective treatment of carbon monoxide poisoning involves splitting the inactivated haemoglobin from carbon monoxide and maintaining adequate tissue oxygenation while this regeneration is in progress. Both requirements depend on supplemental oxygen administration. At high enough concentrations, oxygen displaces bound carbon monoxide from haemoglobin and also, as discussed above, dissolved plasma oxygen is sufficient to substitute for haemoglobin carriage. In mild poisoning, these aims can be achieved with inspired 100% oxygen at atmospheric pressure but in severe cases hyperbaric oxygen may be needed. This not only provides more tissue oxygenation but also speeds up carbon monoxide/haemoglobin dissociation.

Q21 For what other therapeutic applications might hyperbaric oxygen be useful?

MCQ ANSWERS AND FEEDBACK

1.E. As resting intrapleural pressure is around −5 mmHg (0.7 kPa) relative to atmospheric pressure, it must be more negative during the rapid thoracic expansion that accompanies a maximal inspiratory effort. Similarly, inspiration must create sub-atmospheric pressure inside the lung. However, since pleural and pulmonary spaces remain separated, absolute intrapleural pressure will always be slightly lower than that in the lung. The values given, with an inspiratory pressure gradient of 75 mmHg or 10 kPa, are only ever achieved with maximally forced inspiration. Even large unforced inspiratory movements usually lower intrapulmonary pressure to only around −30 mmHg (4 kPa).

2.C. We know from the previous question that the maximal pressure gradient that can be created during forced inspiration is around 75 mmHg or 10 kPa. This is equivalent to 1 m of water (the density of mercury is 13.6 times that of water; $13.6 \times 75 = 1020$ mm). It is therefore impossible for the respiratory muscles to expand the chest wall at depths more than around 1 m below the water surface even with maximal inspiratory effort. Breathing through a hose will certainly increase anatomical dead space and absolute resistance to air flow, but the resistance of a 2.5-cm (1-in) hose is trivial over lengths of several feet and the volume of a tube this diameter is only around 450 ml per 1 m length. Such an increase in dead space could be easily compensated for by elevating tidal volume, if the external pressure was not preventing thoracic expansion.

Changes in air density and Po_2 do occur in hyperbaric environments, but are trivial with the 1 atm (101 kPa) change occurring with 1 m descent – and of course Po_2 will rise rather than fall if the absolute barometric pressure rises, since the proportion of oxygen in the air remains constant. The scenario of a free-swimming underwater worker breathing through a hose occurs often in commercial diving but the air needs to be delivered under positive pressure.

3.D. About 2% of the blood ejected from the left ventricle is systemic venous blood from the bronchial and coronary circulations that drains directly into the left heart. As this blood is relatively deoxygenated, it inevitably reduces the Po_2 of the left cardiac output. At resting tidal volume there is as well a small amount of ventilation : perfusion mismatching because the lung is not ventilated evenly.

During exercise, by contrast, the greater lung expansion usually produces almost complete ventilation : perfusion equality. The rate of oxygen diffusion from air to plasma is about three times faster than the rate of blood flow, so there is a large safety margin to ensure equilibration of oxygen in air and plasma even at high cardiac outputs.

4.B. The shape of the oxygen–haemoglobin dissociation curve means there is almost complete saturation of the haemoglobin molecules at all levels of Po_2 greater than 65 mmHg or 8.6 kPa. Appreciable desaturation starts to occur only when the dissolved oxygen tension falls below about 60 mmHg (8 kPa), corresponding to the threshold Po_2 for activation of peripheral chemoreceptors.

5.D. Young sedentary men have maximal oxygen consumptions of around 3 litres/min, which equates to about 45 (ml/min)/kg or 13 METs (metabolic equivalents). A physically fit individual of comparable age would have a Vo_{2max} in the range 55–60 (ml/min)/kg. Only élite aerobic athletes have Vo_{2max} values above 75 (ml/min)/kg. Incidently, despite what you may think intuitively, professional divers are not usually extremely fit in terms of being able to perform high levels of physical work.

6.D. Total lung capacity equals the sum of the volume left in the lung at the end of expiration (the functional residual capacity) and the extra volume that can be added by inspiration (the inspiratory capacity). The residual volume is that volume left in the lung after a maximal expiratory effort – that is, total lung capacity minus forced vital capacity.

7.B. There cannot be an obstructive lung defect because FEV_1: forced vital capacity is greater than 80% and peak expiratory flow is greater than 450 litres/min. However, a total lung capacity of 5 litres and a forced vital capacity of 4.2 litres are very low for a healthy, 184-cm-tall man (expected values around 7 litres and 5.5 litres), suggesting that he has limited ability to inflate his lungs. This cannot be due to respiratory muscle weakness because he can produce normal rates of forced air flow. It is therefore likely that his lungs are stiffer than normal, causing elevated elastic recoil that restricts inspiratory chest expansion. The presence of elevated elastic recoil is also suggested by the rather low 800 ml residual volume (usually 1200–1500 ml for a person of this size). On interview, J.P. revealed that he was an ex-naval diver who had frequently used closed-circuit oxygen-rebreathing apparatus. Chronic exposure to high concentrations of oxygen is known to carry a risk of fibrotic damage to the lung parenchyma.

8. Asthmatic attacks precipitated by exercise are caused by reflex bronchoconstriction following activation of vagal sensory endings in the airways mucosa. The normal function of these endings is to respond to inhaled chemical substances but they are also activated by mucosal drying. The increased ventilatory volume associated with exercise tends to do this, especially if the inhaled air has a low humidity. Close to the water surface the air is extremely humid, so swimming tends not to provoke asthma as much as running does. In scuba diving, however, the air coming from the pressure tank is absolutely dry. It is also cold, which slows down its humidification.

9. Because positive pressure inside the middle ear tends to open the ostium, pressure equilibration usually presents no problem during ascent unless there is pharyngeal inflammation. By contrast, equilibration during descent is difficult without continual swallowing, because increased external pressure tends to collapse the ostium. It will not be possible to open the ostium by voluntary movement below around 1.2 m (4 ft) and eardrum rupture might take place anywhere between 1.3 and 5 m (4–17 ft), indicating that irreversible middle ear damage can easily occur in a supposedly innocuous environment such as a swimming pool.

10.E. The lateral aspect of the tympanic membrane is supplied by the auriculo-temporal branch of the trigeminal and the auricular branch of the vagus, while the medial aspect is supplied by the glossopharyngeal via the tympanic plexus. As well as damage to these nerves initiating vomiting, intractable coughing is also common. This appears to be due specifically to vagal sensory activation.

11.A. If the middle ear is normal, airborne sounds are heard more efficiently than those conducted by bone, because eardrum and ossicular chain amplify airborne vibrations. Therefore, with incomplete impairment of *inner ear* function, the sound of a tuning fork is louder and lasts longer when it is held *in air* near the ear than when it is placed on the mastoid. If the *middle ear* amplification mechanism is damaged, *bone-conducted* sounds become as loud as or even louder than airborne sounds.

Middle ear (*conductive*) deafness commonly occurs as a result of eardrum damage, fixation of the ossicles by otosclerosis, or excessive middle ear pressure due to inflammatory discharge or to foreign liquid. Inner ear (*sensorineural*) deafness is typically caused by damage to the cochlea by barotrauma or excessive noise, or by nerve damage by local ischaemia or emboli. When barometric pressure changes dramatically, it is of course possible for simultaneous disruption of both middle and inner ear functions to occur.

12.B. The masking effect of background noise on hearing acuity is reduced if the amplifier function of the middle ear is impaired. So, with unilateral middle ear deafness, bone-conducted sound is heard more clearly on the affected side.

For both Rinne's test and Weber's test, accurate results depend on using a tuning fork with a relatively high pitch, because low frequency vibration conducted through the bone can be confused with sound. A fork with a pitch of 256 Hz can be used if necessary, but pitches of either 512 Hz or 1024 Hz are preferable.

13.E. Regardless of the absolute solubility of a gas, more will dissolve in body fluids if the barometric pressure increases (that is, if the local concentration of gas molecules increases). At any specific pressure, the volume of dissolved gas takes some time to reach equilibrium. This is partly because of the fact that it has to be distributed via the circulatory system and partly because of different gas solubilities in lipid and water. Nitrogen is 5 times more soluble in fat than in water: therefore lipid-rich tissues take longer to become saturated with this gas especially if, as in synovial capsules and bone marrow, they have a relatively low blood supply.

When a diver ascends too rapidly, gas will come out of solution in tissues or the bloodstream and may disrupt tissue structure or obstruct blood flow. Although this sequence of events happens with both nitrogen and oxygen, oxygen bubbles are usually utilized for local metabolism virtually as they form. By contrast, nitrogen bubbles can be removed only by waiting for them to redissolve as the pressures re-equilibrate. This may take several hours.

14.D. This mixture is equivalent to atmospheric air, which is the standard used for shallow dives. A depth of 6 m (20 ft) increases barometric pressure by only 0.6 atm (60.6 kPa). This is trivial in terms of affecting gas partial pressures although it has significant implications for total gas volumes within tissue spaces.

15.E. At partial pressures higher than 4 atm (404 kPa), nitrogen begins to exert narcotic properties, apparently through the same molecular actions on neuronal membranes as are produced by gaseous anaesthetics. The intensity of nitrogen narcosis increases with depth and divers lose consciousness with ambient P_{N_2} higher than 8 atm (808 kPa). Nitrogen makes up 79% of normal air, so a P_{N_2} of 4 atm (404 kPa) corresponds to a depth of 40 m (130 ft). Ideally, therefore, any dive deeper than this should involve replacing nitrogen by the less toxic gas helium. In practice, if the dive is very brief and only marginally below 40 m (130 ft), most divers would use normal air (option D).

16.I. At inspired partial pressures of oxygen greater than around 1500 mmHg (200 kPa) there is progressive neurological damage due to free radical formation. This pressure equates to that produced when breathing atmospheric air at a depth of 90 m (297 ft) (10 atm). Effective delivery of oxygen to tissues will take place so long as the pulmonary venous P_{O_2} is sufficient to saturate haemoglobin. With a total barometric pressure of 7 atm (707 kPa), 3% oxygen provides an inspired P_{O_2} of $(0.03 \times 7 \times 760)$ or 160 mmHg (21 kPa) – identical to the situation when breathing air at sea level.

At depths of this magnitude, substitution of helium for nitrogen also has substantial advantages. As discussed above, it lacks the toxic effects of nitrogen. A second advantage is that helium is seven times less dense than nitrogen, so the work of breathing highly compressed gas is much reduced. A third potential benefit is that, because helium is less soluble in body fluids than nitrogen, it may reduce the time needed for decompression during ascent. In practice, there appears to be little difference in the decompression requirements. One drawback of helium is that its thermal conductivity is much greater than that of nitrogen. This exaggerates dehydration of the airways mucosa and also predisposes the diver to hypothermia.

The need for different gas mixtures at different barometric pressures requires divers to change from one mixture to another as they submerge, using cylinders that have been dropped to appropriate depths. This increases the complexity of maintaining the gas supply and of arranging the decompression schedule. Because the oxygen mixture used at 60 m (190 ft) would provide a Po_2 of only 39 mmHg (5.2 kPa) at 6 m (20 ft) and 30 mmHg (4 kPa) at 3 m (10 ft), which are the longest duration decompression staging points, at least one change of gas is needed during ascent.

17.D. Boyle's law defines the relationship between gas pressure and gas volume as a reciprocal one. With halving of pressure from 2 atm to 1 atm (202–101 kPa), the volume of gas must double.

18.A. Decreased Po_2 and increased Pco_2 in the airways cause bronchodilation, as part of a protective mechanism that will reduce resistance to air flow in poorly ventilated areas of lung. Similarly, elevated Po_2 and lower Pco_2 will cause bronchoconstriction. Since inspired air at 10 m (2 atm) has a Po_2 of 300 mmHg (40 kPa) there will be a generalized increase of airways resistance and this will increase the likelihood of air trapping.

19. No carbon monoxide is present in normal air.

20. At 60 m (190 ft) (7 atm) depth, partial pressures of both carbon monoxide and oxygen are increased seven-fold above their values at sea level. The inspired carbon monoxide level is therefore 0.1 mmHg rather than 0.015 mmHg, enough to displace oxygen from around 30% of the haemoglobin binding sites.

At depth, this deficit in oxygen carriage is masked by the simultaneous increase in Po_2, which also increases seven-fold. So instead of only 0.3 ml of oxygen being dissolved in every 100 ml plasma, the solubility is 2.1 ml oxygen/100 ml, providing transport of 105 ml oxygen/min at a cardiac output of 5 litres/min. Together with the 70% residual capacity of haemoglobin to bind oxygen, this is able to maintain the diver's metabolic needs as long as the ambient pressure is high. On ascent, however, dissolved oxygen falls back to negligible levels while the haemoglobin remains inactive.

The presence of the carboxyhaemoglobin complex also explains the mismatch between a relatively high proportion of oxyhaemoglobin and the severity of hypoxia. Occupancy of some haemoglobin-binding sites by carbon monoxide increases the affinity for oxygen of any remaining sites. In consequence, the dissociation curve is shifted dramatically to the right and much less oxygen than usual is unloaded in the tissue capillaries.

21. Breathing oxygen at high partial pressure causes more oxygen to be dissolved in the plasma, so this is potentially useful for treatment of any condition that involves inadequate oxygen delivery to the tissues. Hyperbaric oxygen can be used for emergency treatment of patients in whom there is extreme anaemia, for instance following massive haemolysis. It is also valuable in patients with anaerobic bacterial infections such as caused by *Clostridia* (gas gangrene), because these strains of bacteria are not able to survive in the presence of high oxygen tensions.

CASE REVIEW

Understanding the physical and physiological changes that accompany altered ambient pressure helps in interpreting a variety of clinical scenarios, in particular with regard to respiratory disease. Furthermore, the individual physician is becoming more and more likely to see patients with specific dysfunctions related to pressurization and decompression. Not only are there large populations of professional divers, caisson workers and pilots throughout the world, but over 800 000 new scuba divers are certificated every year.

The changes in nitrogen solubility that accompany entry to and exit from hyperbaric environments also occur with altitudes above sea level but, because of the small absolute changes in pressure relative to those in water, alterations sufficient to cause decompression sickness are not common. For instance, if a commercial aircraft flying at the normal altitude of around 10 000 m (33 000 ft) lost cabin pressure completely, passengers would be exposed to a barometric pressure of around 240 mmHg (32 kPa). This would cause severe hypoxia, as the ambient Po_2 would be only 21% × 240 or 50 mmHg (6.7 kPa). But since the absolute pressure would have fallen by less than 1 atm (101 kPa), there would be only a negligible change in nitrogen solubility.

Carbon monoxide poisoning is relatively common because the gas is generated as a by-product of fossil fuel combustion and because the early stages of intoxication are usually symptomless. Breathing air with a low oxygen content stimulates peripheral chemoreceptors and respiratory drive, leading to dyspnoea. However, dissolved oxygen levels are not affected by carbon monoxide, so there is no chemoreceptor activation and no warning of the imminent fall in oxygen carriage.

The carboxyhaemoglobin complex has a slightly pinker colour than oxyhaemoglobin and this has led to statements in some textbooks that victims of carbon monoxide poisoning have a cherry-red appearance. In practice, this is rarely seen except *post mortem* and almost all victims who are alive have normal skin colour.

Theoretically, hyperbaric oxygen therapy could be used in a variety of conditions where tissue damage is caused by poor local blood supply, such as diabetes and stroke. Nevertheless, clinical trials have not indicated any consistent clinical benefit. This might be due to interference by a second effect of oxygen. You will remember that tissue hypoxia causes local vasodilation – an important way of matching regional perfusion to metabolic needs. The opposite is also true, so hyperoxia causes vasoconstriction. It is possible that, by limiting tissue perfusion and oxygen delivery, this constrictor effect may have masked any beneficial actions of hyperoxia in the diabetes and stroke trials.

KEY POINTS

- Underwater, ambient pressure increases by 1 atm (760 mmHg, 101 kPa) per 10 m (33 ft) depth.
- This has significant implications for respiratory work and for gas volumes within the body.
- When air is trapped within tissue spaces such as the ear or lung, the volume changes produced underwater can cause tissue rupture at depths as little as 1–2 m (3–6 ft).

- At ambient pressures of more than 3 atm (303 kPa), the elevated partial pressures of oxygen and nitrogen begin to exert significant effects. Both gases impair neurological function.
- The increased tissue solubility of nitrogen at high partial pressures requires slow reduction in pressure during ascent to avoid bubbles forming in blood and tissues.

ADDITIONAL READING

Bove AA (2004) *Bove and Davis' Diving Medicine*, 4th edition. WB Saunders Co., Philadelphia.

Dean JB, Mulkey DK, Garcia AJ III, Putnam RW & Henderson RA III (2003) Neuronal sensitivity to hyperoxia, hypercapnia, and inert gases at hyperbaric pressures. *Journal of Applied Physiology* **95**: 883–909.

DeGorordo A, Vallejo-Manzur F, Chanin K & Varon J (2003) Diving emergencies. *Resuscitation* **59**: 171–80.

Emerson G (2004) The dilemma of managing carbon monoxide poisoning. *Emergency Medicine Australasia* **16**: 101–2.

Hamilton-Farrell M & Bhattacharyya A (2004) Barotrauma. *Injury* **35**: 359–70.

Breathing difficulties after insect bite and air travel

CASE AND MCQS

Case introduction

F.B. is a healthy 36-year-old woman who has travelled to New Zealand from her home in England to visit relatives. She is brought by car to an Auckland accident and emergency department by her partner.

About 15 minutes earlier, she had been playing ball with her children and was stung on the forearm by a bee. Within a few minutes, she began to feel light-headed, nauseous and 'uneasy'. She then found it difficult to take a deep breath and it felt as though her throat was closing up.

On examination, Ms B. appears very anxious, is sweating and is taking rapid shallow breaths. Her temperature is 37.0°C; her heart rate is 110 beats/min; her arterial blood pressure is 80/40 mmHg and her respiratory rate is 20 breaths/min.

Auscultation of her chest shows normal heart sounds with no evidence of cardiac murmurs; her radial and brachial pulses are weak and thready. There are bilateral inspiratory and expiratory wheezes together with some supraclavicular retraction during inspiration.

Her skin is warm and flushed. There is no peripheral cyanosis. On being questioned, she says that she has been stung by bees in the past but that this had produced only a local redness and a small swelling that disappeared quickly.

| Q1 | List the important cardiovascular symptoms that are present. |

| Q2 | List the important respiratory symptoms that are present. |

These symptoms are characteristic of an allergic (anaphylactic) response to a bee sting. The response is due to the production of allergen-specific antibodies produced as a result of an earlier sting but they are often not activated until after multiple stings.

Before we proceed, let us make sure that you remember some basics of the immune response. Answer questions 3–7 using options from the following list:

A. IgA antibodies
B. IgD antibodies
C. IgE antibodies
D. IgG antibodies
E. IgM antibodies

| Q3 | Are the most abundant class of blood-borne antibody. |

| Q4 | Are present in most exocrine secretions. |

| Q5 | Act as the receptor for antigen binding on B cell membranes. |

| Q6 | Help protect against infestation by parasitic worms. |

| Q7 | Mediate allergic responses to insect venoms. |

Q8 The antibodies involved in allergic responses are produced by:

A. B-lymphocytes
B. T-lymphocytes
C. eosinophils
D. basophils
E. neutrophils

Q9 The final mediators of the allergic response are released when the antibody docks on and activates:

A. enterochromaffin cells
B. mast cells
C. endothelial cells
D. adrenocortical cells
E. none of the above

Q10 This activation stimulates the release of:

A. histamine
B. leukotrienes
C. prostaglandins
D. all of the above
E. only A and B above

Q11 Collectively, the these mediators will produce:

A. pulmonary oedema
B. peripheral oedema
C. decreased peripheral resistance
D. all of the above
E. none of the above

Q12 The respiratory effects of these mediators will be:

A. decreased work of breathing
B. increased airway resistance
C. increased alveolar exchange area
D. decreased airway resistance
E. both B and C above

Now back to the patient, who is very ill. The physician's actions have to be aimed at alleviating the effects of these mediators.
- First, she is given oxygen via a nasal mask.
- Adrenaline (epinephrine) is given subcutaneously (0.5 ml of 1:1000 or 0.5 mg in an adult).
- A beta-adrenoreceptor agonist such as albuterol (salbutamol) is given by nebulizer.
- It is also usual practice to provide plasma volume expansion with infused colloid (1–2 litres intravenously).

Q13 Adrenaline (epinephrine) is likely to be beneficial because it causes:

A. bronchodilation
B. peripheral vasoconstriction
C. increased cardiac contractility
D. all of the above
E. both A and C above

Q14 What other types of drug do you think might be useful?

Within 15–20 minutes of commencing treatment, Ms B. begins to feel much better. She can breathe much more easily, her wheezes have diminished markedly to a slight one in the expiratory phase and the supraclavicular retractions have disappeared.

Her blood pressure is now 119/73 mmHg, her heart rate is down to 61 beats/min and her skin is clear.

She is given another two albuterol nebulizer treatments, is held overnight in hospital on low doses of prednisolone and diphenhydramine, and is discharged the next day.

The following week she flies home to Europe, changing planes in Los Angeles. The total flight time for the two legs of her trip is around 23 hours. Ten days after her return she wakes up in the middle of the night with a sharp left-sided pain in the chest and some difficulty in breathing. She is able to get back to sleep again but when she wakes in the morning the pain is much stronger and more persistent, and is even worse when she tries to take a deep breath. She finds that she becomes quite short of breath when she walks downstairs to the kitchen and back to her bedroom again. Concerned, she comes to you as her family doctor.

Examination shows an apparently healthy woman with mild breathlessness (*dyspnoea*). She is a smoker (16 cigarettes/day) and appears bright and alert. She has not had any recent infections, back pain or abdominal pain. The only health-related event she has noticed since the episode of anaphylaxis in New Zealand is that her right calf has felt sore during the time she has been home.

She has slight tachycardia (96 beats/min); her blood pressure is 118/67 mmHg; her respiratory rate is 16 breaths/min.

Her mouth and pharynx are clear and she has indication of swollen lymph nodes (*adenopathy*). Her jugular venous pressure appears to be normal. Chest examination indicates a normal regular cardiac rhythm without any murmurs. Her radial and pedal pulses are full and seemed normal bilaterally.

Her chest sounds indicate that the lungs are clear on both sides though there is a slight grating when she inspires deeply. Her chest wall is not tender, nor is her abdomen. There is slight pitting oedema on her right foot and ankle and her right calf is mildly tender and slightly swollen.

Q15 At this stage of investigation, Ms B.'s problems seem likely to involve a defect in which of the following systems?

A. cardiovascular
B. respiratory or cardiovascular
C. renal or cardiovascular
D. neuromuscular, renal or cardiovascular
E. neuromuscular, cardiovascular or respiratory

Electrocardiography shows sinus tachycardia, with evidence of blockade of the right bundle branch (Fig. 4.1).

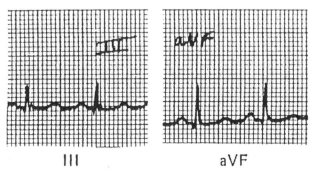

Fig. 4.1 ECG records from leads II and aVF in patient F.B. on initial examination.

Q16 The characteristics of the records in Fig. 4.1 that indicate right bundle branch block are:

A. ventricular depolarization time greater than 200 ms and Q wave present
B. ventricular depolarization time greater than 200 ms and no Q wave
C. ventricular depolarization time greater than 100 ms and Q wave present
D. ventricular depolarization time greater than 100 ms and no Q wave
E. ventricular depolarization time normal but R wave inverted

You send Ms B. for blood tests, chest X-ray and blood gas assessment and take a sputum sample for culture.

Of the potential problems that may exist, myocardial infarction and pulmonary embolism are likely to be the most threatening in the short term. Myocardial infarction may result in serious arrhythmias, ventricular muscle dysfunction, circulatory collapse and death. A pulmonary embolus, if untreated, may lead to progressive clot formation, pulmonary ischaemia, circulatory collapse and death. Most pulmonary embolic episodes result from clots that had formed in a lower limb (deep vein thrombosis; DVT).

The obvious and easily available investigations may not give unequivocal answers. Chest X-ray has low sensitivity and specificity for pulmonary embolism. Over 30% of patients with an embolus have a normal chest X-ray; another 30% will have an infiltrate that resembles pneumonia. In relation to the electrocardiogram, some definite changes would be expected if myocardial infarction is involved but not necessarily in the case of pulmonary embolism.

The electrocardiogram shows only tachycardia and right bundle branch blockade, consistent with but not indicative of infarction. The chest X-ray, when received, shows no overt lung pathology. Blood and sputum tests are also negative, tending to rule out several potential problems including an infarct and pneumonia.

This leaves pulmonary embolism as the prime suspect, so you decide to ask for some tests of ventilation/perfusion efficiency. Before looking at the result, it will be useful to examine some of the physiology of ventilation/perfusion relationships in the normal lung.

Ventilation of the alveoli is achieved by their periodic inflation and deflation with atmospheric air. There is a substantial part of the respiratory tree where there is no gas exchange. This includes the trachea and bronchi and some areas of the lung parenchyma.

Q17 The region of lung in which there is inadequate gas exchange is collectively termed:

A. anatomical dead space
B. residual volume
C. physiological dead space
D. alveolar space
E. none of the above

The action of ventilation flushes out residual air, replacing it with new air. With uniform ventilation, all alveoli are flushed at the same rate but if some parts are not ventilated adequately then the gas they contain will have a different composition and appear more slowly in the exhaled air.

Q18 One test that determines the normality of ventilation/perfusion ratio is called:

A. the breath-sampling technique
B. the multiple breath washout
C. the oxygen breathing test
D. the ventilation test
E. none of the above

For efficient functioning of the lung it is important that alveolar ventilation (V) should match the regional blood flow (Q). Poor local flow will have little capacity for carrying respiratory gases and gives rise to physiological dead space. Conversely, flow through regions of low ventilation is equally inefficient, acting as a shunt. Smooth muscle in the pulmonary arterioles constricts when the local intra-alveolar air contains low oxygen levels and this diverts blood away from underventilated areas.

Gravity also has an effect on the distribution of pulmonary blood flow. When a person is upright there is an approximately 24 cmH$_2$O (19 mmHg) difference between the apex and base of the lungs. When standing upright, both ventilation and perfusion therefore change – the latter more than the former. Ventilation/perfusion (V/Q) ratios express the degree of matching of ventilation and perfusion. Figure 4.2 illustrates the matching of ventilation and perfusion along the length of an upright lung, together with the equivalent V/Q ratios.

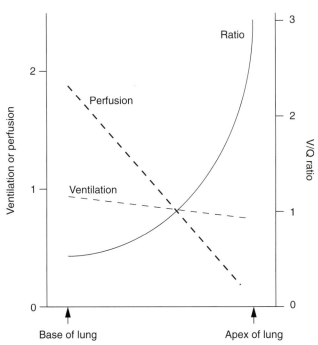

Fig. 4.2 Distribution of ventilation and perfusion in a normal lung, in a standing individual.

As well as the oxygen breath test, you arrange for Ms B. to have a ventilation/perfusion scan, in an effort to localize any areas of inefficient V/Q matching. This scan involves simultaneous imaging of regional ventilation using inhaled xenon-133 and regional perfusion using technetium-99m-labelled albumin.

The results of both these tests are equivocal in that they do not show clear signs of a mismatch, although the scan indicates some small ventilated areas where there is possibly low perfusion. Lack of definitive results with these tests is not surprising if the area of disturbance is small or diffuse. However, you are still concerned about a potential embolus, so you decide to look specifically at the soreness in her leg with an ultrasonic scan around the area of soreness, together with further blood tests to see if her clotting mechanisms are in some way enhanced.

Q19 A suitable test to determine abnormality of clotting mechanisms would be:

A. prothrombin time
B. bleeding time
C. thromboplastin time
D. A and C above
E. all of the above

The ultrasound scan indicates a substantial clot in the popliteal vein. From this finding, there is a distinct possibility that a subsidiary clot has detached itself from the main one and lodged in the capillaries of the lung. There may be multiple small intrapulmonary clots. The results of the new blood tests are clear evidence of her blood being hypercoagulable, with prothrombin and thromboplastin times that are both slightly shorter than normal.

On this basis, you decide to administer heparin to reduce the chances of further clotting. You continue the anticoagulation with warfarin. The anticoagulant effects of both drugs need to be closely monitored and specifically titrated to ensure that the chances of subsequent clots are minimized. A useful target is to maintain the prothrombin time at about 1.5–2 times normal.

Since heparin and warfarin will only prevent further clot formation, some consideration could be given to the use of thrombolytic agents which actively dissolve existing clots over a period. Either streptokinase or urokinase are suitable, though the former can be antigenic. This has the implication that the dosage of subsequent administrations of streptokinase may have to be adjusted upwards to provide inactivation of circulating antibodies.

After 3 days of this treatment, Ms B.'s symptoms are much diminished and she is allowed to go home, with instructions to take the oral anticoagulant warfarin until further notice. She is cautioned against taking aspirin during this period.

Q20 Why might aspirin be contraindicated in a patient being treated with an anticoagulant drug?

MCQ ANSWERS AND FEEDBACK

1. Her arterial blood pressure is low and her heart rate is high. Her heart seems normal. Her peripheral circulation suggests some dilatation of blood vessels.

2. Her respiration is shallow and fast. The respiratory wheezes indicate difficulty in moving air in and out of her lungs, suggesting bronchoconstriction.

3.D. In a normal individual around 75% of the total serum antibodies are IgG.

4.A. IgA immunoglobulins are present in tears, milk and mucous secretions of the gastrointestinal, respiratory and genitourinary tracts.

5.E. The IgM immunoglobulins are secreted in the early stages of the plasma cell response.

6.C. Despite their biological importance, IgE constitute only around 0.01% of the total serum antibodies.

7.C. IgE antibodies mediate all allergic responses to foreign proteins.

8.A. The T-lymphocyte is involved in cell-mediated immunity, not antibody-mediated immunity. None of the other leukocyte types is involved in the initial stage of immune reactions.

9.B. The antibodies bind to mast cells and basophils. Mast cells are found throughout the body and are most frequent in the lungs, skin and gut. As well as being involved in allergic responses, they also have a role in fighting infections. Activation of circulating basophils enhances the systemic response to allergic stimuli.

10.D. The IgE molecules stimulate degranulation of mast cells, which causes release of the preformed mediators. These include histamine, prostaglandins, leukotrienes and platelet-activating factor.

11.D. Following the release of these mediators in large amounts, widespread vasodilatation is evoked though relaxation of vascular smooth muscle: they also directly induce an increase in capillary permeability. The latter will affect both systemic and pulmonary capillaries and so influence gas transport at both sites.

12.B. The anaphylactic mediators are potent constrictors of bronchial smooth muscle and also cause inflammation of the bronchial mucosa.

13.D. Adrenaline (epinephrine) will act on the cardiac muscle and smooth muscle in the bronchi through a beta-agonist action, and on the vascular smooth muscle in the peripheral circulation via an alpha-adrenoreceptor agonist action.

14. Antagonists at histamine-1 receptors such as diphenhydramine will reduce the histamine-mediated cardiorespiratory problems and the anti-inflammatory actions of glucocorticoids such as prednisolone will reduce all the pro-inflammatory effects of the allergic mediators. The action of glucocorticoids has a latency of several hours, so it is important to provide immediate treatment along the other lines indicated.

15.E. The symptoms are consistent with the following: cardiovascular – acute myocardial infarct and pericarditis; respiratory – spontaneous pneumothorax, pulmonary embolism, pneumonia, pleurisy; neuromuscular – intercostal muscle damage, damage to costal cartilage. There is nothing to suggest that a pleuretic chest pain and dyspnoea are likely to originate from renal problems.

16.C. Under the conditions of right bundle branch block, no conduction occurs down the right bundle branch. The septum is depolarized from the left side as usual, causing a normal Q wave but widening of the whole QRS waveform because right ventricular depolarization has to occur by intermuscle fibre conduction from the left ventricle. With complete branch block the QRS duration is 100–140 ms rather than the normal 60–70 ms. The particular record obtained from Ms B. and shown in Fig. 4.1 shows a QRS of around 110 ms.

17.C. Physiological dead space includes those parts of the conducting airway tree that are not capable of gas exchange, i.e. the anatomical dead space of the trachea, bronchi and bronchioles, together with those alveoli that are not adequately perfused or are not adequately ventilated. The latter component is frequently increased in volume by disease states.

18.C. In this test, the patient breathes pure oxygen and the expired air is analysed for the fraction of nitrogen in each successive breath. The nitrogen percentage is plotted against the breath number. The nitrogen is derived from the breaths before starting the oxygen. If the lungs are being ventilated efficiently and uniformly the plot is a normal exponential. If ventilation is inefficient and non-uniform the nitrogen is washed out more slowly and the plot falls slowly. Gravity, smooth muscle control of airway diameter and age all influence the normal distribution of ventilation in the lungs; disease has additional effects.

19.D. Thromboplastin time measures the integrity of intrinsic and common pathways, while prothrombin time assesses the extrinsic and common pathways.

20. Aspirin inhibits the activity of cyclo-oxygenase-2, which is essential for platelet aggregation. It therefore potentiates the anticoagulant effect of drugs such as warfarin, leading to increased risk of unwanted bleeding.

CASE REVIEW

Anaphylaxis is a frightening experience for both patient and doctor. The sudden onset and nature of the symptoms are striking and centre around the great difficulties that a previously healthy patient has in breathing. If rapid and appropriate action is not taken the patient will rapidly become severely hypoxic and hypotensive, and die. The bronchial constriction and oedema of the bronchial tree increase greatly the resistance to inspiratory and expiratory efforts and interfere with the access of inspired air to the alveoli and the expiration of exhaled air. Blood gas exchange is therefore greatly compromised. The effect of a subcutaneous injection of adrenaline (epinephrine) is dramatic and an important lifesaver.

A summary of the processes involved are shown in Fig. 4.3.

Anaphylactic reactions can be induced by a wide range of agents. They include insect bites and stings, and allergic responses to various foods such as shellfish and nuts are common. A common reaction is that provoked by penicillin, which accounts for many cases in the UK and USA.

Ms B.'s second episode turned out to be pulmonary embolus as a consequence of a deep vein thrombosis (DVT). The predisposing factors for DVT are relative stasis of blood for some time – typically due to sitting or lying for a considerable period without much muscle movement, increased coagulability of the blood and vessel wall abnormalities in the large veins. It is only rarely due to a specific abnormality in haematological clotting mechanisms. Frequently, the affected leg is swollen and oedematous. The pulmonary consequences are potentially dangerous and need to be guarded against even when there is no evidence of a clot in the lung.

A patient who has suffered a DVT should be advised to cease smoking and to avoid taking oral contraceptives, as both are known risk factors. The evidence that DVT is likely to follow a long journey by air is presently equivocal, but it is sensible to take measures that will minimize the risk. Thus on a long journey, whether by air, rail or bus, it is sensible to move around periodically and to mobilize the leg and thigh

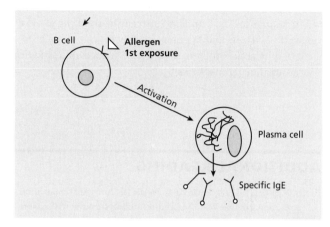

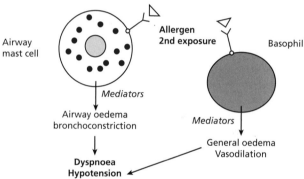

Fig. 4.3 Summary of the processes involved in allergic shock. The shaded upper panel represents events occurring on initial exposure to the allergen and the lower panel shows the consequences of subsequent exposure.

muscles with specific exercises. The arrangement of the seats and back support may slow the flow of blood in the larger muscles of the calf and thighs. Movement and muscle contractions mitigate this. Tight stockings clearly assist as well by reducing the venous congestion that can occur under these circumstances.

KEY POINTS

- Anaphylaxis to bee sting is a type 1 hypersensitivity response requiring previous sensitization.
- It involves IgE-mediated activation of mast cells and basophils resulting in release of histamine, leukotrienes, prostaglandins and platelet-activating factor.
- These mediators cause increased vascular permeability, vasodilation and bronchoconstriction, resulting in respiratory distress and hypotensive shock.
- Anaphylactic shock is fatal if not treated quickly with adrenaline (epinephrine).
- Chest pain and dyspnoea are diffuse symptoms with multiple potential causes, and differential diagnosis is needed, especially between acute myocardial infarction and pulmonary embolus.
- Pulmonary emboli are caused commonly by deep vein thrombosis.
- Risk factors for deep vein thrombosis include smoking, oral contraceptives, hypercoagulability of blood and prolonged immobility.

ADDITIONAL READING

Brown SG, Wiese MD, Blackman KE & Heddle RJ (2003) Ant venom immunotherapy: a double-blind, placebo-controlled, crossover trial. *Lancet* **361**: 1001–6.

Gorman WP, Davis KR & Donnelly R (2000) Swollen lower limb-1: general assessment and deep vein thrombosis. *British Medical Journal* **320**: 1453–6.

Hughes RJ, Hopkins RJ, Hill S *et al.* (2003) Frequency of venous thromboembolism in low to moderate risk long distance air travellers: the New Zealand Air Traveller's Thrombosis (NZATT) study. *Lancet* **362**: 2039–44.

McLean-Tooke AP, Bethune CA, Fay AC & Spickett GP (2003) Adrenaline in the treatment of anaphylaxis: what is the evidence? *British Medical Journal* **327**: 1332–5.

Roitt IM (2001) *Essential Immunology*, 10th edition, Blackwell Science, Oxford.

Infertility in a female athlete

CASE AND MCQS

Case introduction

Ms K.L. is a thin (height 170 cm (5 ft, 7 in), weight 55 kg (121 lb), BMI 19.0), healthy-looking woman aged 25. Her blood pressure (sitting) is 110/60 mmHg and her pulse rate is 48 beats/min.

She is a physiotherapist who has enjoyed good health all her life, except for a bout of German measles at the age of 10. She has been a long-distance runner since her early teens, and has been involved regularly in high-level competition since the age of 15. She was picked for the national team in an international competition last year, but had to withdraw due to a stress fracture of the ankle incurred some weeks before the event. She has been married to a fellow physiotherapist (also aged 25) for a year and they have been trying to have a baby since then, without success.

Her periods commenced when she was 15 years old. In general, they have been regular, with a cycle length over the last few years of about 24 days. However, she has noticed that during times of intense pre-competition training she sometimes misses a period altogether. This has contributed to the stress surrounding her failure to become pregnant. She does not experience premenstrual pain.

One obvious reason for her failure to conceive would be absence of ovulation. You can easily obtain some information on whether ovulation occurs by determining how basal body temperature varies during the ovarian cycle. You discuss with Ms L. the procedures for taking and recording her basal body temperature accurately, using an oral thermometer. You emphasize the need to maintain daily records and also to take measurements on waking, so that her temperature is not elevated by physical or mental activity.

Q1 Existence of normal ovulation can be confirmed by:

A. sustained reduction of body temperature during the second half of the cycle
B. brief elevation of body temperature coinciding with ovulation
C. sustained elevation of body temperature during the second half of the cycle
D. brief depression of body temperature coinciding with ovulation
E. sustained elevation of body temperature during the menstrual phase

Q2 The change in body temperature during the ovarian cycle is due to secretion of:

A. luteinizing hormone (LH)
B. oestrogens
C. chorionic gonadotrophin
D. progesterone
E. cortisol

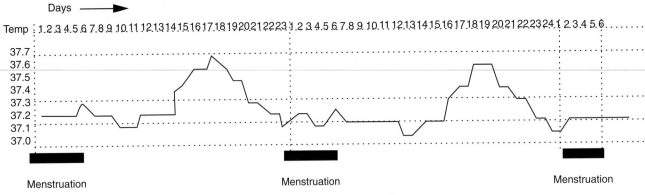

Days ⟶

Temp 1.2.3.4.5.6.7.8.9.10.11.12.13.14.15.16.17.18.19.20.21.22.23.1.2.3.4.5.6.7.8.9.10.11.12.13.14.15.16.17.18.19.20.21.22.23.24.1.2.3.4.5.6.........

Menstruation   Menstruation   Menstruation

Fig. 5.1 Two-month daily temperature chart returned by K.L., showing the days of menstruation.

Nine weeks later, Ms L. brings back her last two months' temperature charts, which are shown in Fig. 5.1.

Q3 On the basis of these records, Ms L.'s cycle:

A. is anovulatory
B. is ovulatory but the luteal phase is abnormally short
C. is ovulatory but no corpus luteum is formed
D. is ovulatory but the luteal phase is abnormally long
E. is normal

So you now have evidence that Ms L. is ovulating but that she has abnormal corpus luteum function.

Q4 The corpus luteum:

A. inhibits further ovulation
B. stimulates endometrial angiogenesis
C. stimulates endometrial glandular growth
D. all of the above
E. none of the above

Q5 The normal process of implantation and placentation is prevented by a short luteal phase because it takes more than 7 days after fertilization of the ovum for:

A. development of the fertilized ovum into a morula
B. formation of adequate endometrial glycogen stores for implantation
C. passage of the fertilized egg along the oviduct
D. creation of a nutritive environment in the uterus
E. vascularization of the decidua

Considering the patient's history and the data that you have on her hormonal status, you are now in a position to decide how to help her become pregnant. What will your next move be?

Q6 Should you:

A. arrange hormone assays to determine whether ovulation occurs?
B. arrange a progesterone assay to confirm luteal function?
C. advise her to reduce her athletic commitments?
D. advise her to undertake psychotherapy?
E. advise her to have intercourse 2 days before the calculated day of ovulation?

Ms L. agrees to follow your advice and, eight months later, she comes to consult you again. She virtually stopped training shortly after you last discussed the problem. For the last seven months, she has restricted her exercise to a 2-km jogging session daily. During the last few months, her cycle length has lengthened to 28–29 days and menstrual blood loss has increased noticeably.

She has continued to monitor her basal body temperature daily, and last month's chart shows a luteal phase commencing 14 days before menstruation. Her last period was due 8–9 days prior to her current visit, so she wonders if she is now pregnant.

Q7 If she is pregnant (estimated 21 days post-fertilization), this could be confirmed by:

A. detection of urinary oestrogen
B. detection of urinary prolactin
C. detection of urinary chorionic gonadotrophin (hCG)
D. detection of urinary progesterone
E. no urinary markers until at least 28 days post fertilization

Q8 Secretion of hCG by the placenta during early pregnancy is important in order to:

A. convert fetal dihydroepiandrosterone (DHEA) into oestrogen
B. stimulate gonadal steroid production
C. suppress pituitary LH secretion
D. maintain the endometrium
E. all of the above

Q9 As well as this function, plasma hCG during the first two months of gestation is essential for:

A. activation of Leydig cells in the male fetus
B. regression of Müllerian ducts in the male fetus
C. regression of Wolffian ducts in the female fetus
D. descent of testes in the male fetus
E. all of the above

Q10 The roles of circulating progesterone during pregnancy include:

A. protecting the fetus from infection
B. stimulating plasma protein production
C. stimulating mammary duct development
D. upregulating expression of mammary enzymes
E. all of the above

Q11 The roles of circulating oestrogens during pregnancy include:

A. inhibiting uterine contractility by breaking down gap junctions
B. inducing myometrial progesterone receptors
C. stimulating mammary duct development
D. inhibiting gonadotrophin-releasing hormone (GnRH) secretion
E. all of the above

Q12 By 10 weeks gestation, the corpus luteum no longer functions as a major source of oestrogen because by this time:

A. the corpus luteum has degenerated
B. corpus luteal stores of precursor cholesterol are exhausted
C. the fetal adrenal cortex is mature
D. fetal capacity to synthesize cholesterol has risen
E. the placenta is able to synthesize DHEA

Not surprisingly for a first-time mother who has had difficulty conceiving, Ms L. is very concerned about her ability to carry her baby to term. You therefore agree to place her in a programme that will monitor her endocrine and cardiovascular status as pregnancy progresses.

Q13 The maternal plasma hormone of choice for assessing fetal viability is:

A. DHEA
B. chorionic somatomammotrophin (hCS)
C. progesterone
D. oestriol
E. oestradiol

Over the next 6 months, Ms L.'s steroid profiles are as expected and her blood pressure is stable at 120/76 mmHg. The next report that you receive, however, indicates that, at gestational age 36 weeks, oestrogen production is rather less than expected (Fig. 5.2) and that blood pressure has risen somewhat.

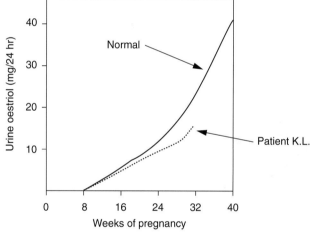

Fig. 5.2 Pattern of normal oestriol production during pregnancy and the data obtained for K.L.

You ask her to come into your office next day for an assessment. On examination, you find that she has a blood pressure (sitting) of 150/95 mmHg and a pulse rate of 84 beats/min. She has pitting oedema of the ankles and a urine sample shows protein on dipstick analysis. You advise her to rest as much as possible and continue to monitor her cardiovascular, renal and hormonal status closely. Over the next week:

- plasma oestriol rises only about half as much as expected
- fetal heart rate rises from 90 to 115 beats/min
- maternal blood pressure rises to 160/100 mmHg
- proteinuria becomes more severe.

These changes are characteristic of a syndrome called pre-eclampsia and together indicate progressive maternal renal damage (proteinuria, water retention, hypertension) as well as serious fetal growth retardation (low oestriol) and fetal hypoxia (fetal tachycardia). If this situation continues, fetal death is inevitable, and the mother may suffer irreversible damage to her kidneys and possibly sustain a cerebrovascular haemorrhage (stroke).

It is decided to induce labour.

Q14 In normal labour at term, the initiating stimulus for uterine contraction is:

A. a rise in the maternal plasma progesterone : oestrogen ratio
B. release of maternal oxytocin
C. release of maternal cortisol
D. release of uterine prostaglandin
E. none of the above

Q15 At 37 weeks gestation, labour could be induced by maternal infusion of:

A. vasopressin (antidiuretic hormone)
B. oxytocin
C. a beta$_2$-adrenoreceptor stimulant
D. prostaglandin E
E. either B or D

Q16 If the baby is born three weeks prematurely, this will mean that all its organ systems must cope with the extrauterine environment before the end of normal development. The factor for which this is most likely to create problems is:

A. alveolar type I cell function
B. antibody production
C. thermoregulation
D. neural control of respiration
E. renal tubular function

Ms L. is admitted to the maternity unit and labour is induced. Delivery proceeds uneventfully and the baby is placed in a humidicrib. The infant is a male, body weight 2.3 kg (5 lb) (expected weight at 37 weeks around 2.9 kg (6 lb)). He is vigorous and active, with normal pulses. He has a slight systolic murmur, which is not pronounced enough to be an immediate concern. Blood pressure by auscultation is recorded as 100/55 mmHg and pulse rate is 90 beats/min. Respiratory rate is 18 breaths/min.

Ms L. would like to feed baby L. while he is in the humidicrib and collection of breast milk is attempted with a suction pump. However, although her breasts are engorged, no milk can be collected.

Q17 Lack of milk ejection despite the presence of milk secretion may involve:

A. defective secretion of oxytocin
B. defective secretion of prolactin
C. defective secretion of hCS
D. defective secretion of hypothalamic GnRH
E. absence of oestrogen-mediated mammary duct development

The psychological problems that are often seen in primiparous mothers separated from their infants can be alleviated by allowing them to handle the baby. Using this strategy, Ms L. is expelling adequate breast milk by 24 hours after birth.

However, at this time baby L. is not feeding well and is restless and crying. His blood pressure is now 110/50 mmHg, pulse rate is 100 beats/min, respiratory rate is 24 breaths/min and his skin is pale. His systolic murmur is more pronounced. A catheter is passed through his right heart into his pulmonary artery and the following data are collected:

Right atrial pressure	3/0 mmHg
Right ventricular pressure	40/0 mmHg
Pulmonary arterial pressure	40/28 mmHg
Pulmonary wedge pressure	12/6 mmHg
Right atrial P_{O_2}	40 mmHg (5.3 kPa)
Right atrial P_{CO_2}	46 mmHg (6.1 kPa)
Arterial P_{O_2}	96 mmHg (12.8 kPa)
Arterial P_{CO_2}	30 mmHg (4.0 kPa)
Arterial pH	7.28
Haemoglobin	15 g/100 ml
Haematocrit	45%

Q18 Recorded values for which of the following parameters are unexpected?

A. systemic arterial pressure
B. right ventricular pressure
C. pulmonary arterial pressure
D. pulmonary wedge pressure
E. all of the above

Q19 From these data, baby L.'s acidosis and distress are likely to involve:

A. defective ventilation
B. defective gas exchange
C. defective pulmonary blood flow
D. defective systemic blood flow
E. none of the above; they all appear normal

In a neonate, the most obvious causes of this type of problem to consider are those related to abnormal development or failure of the normal adjustments from fetal to extrauterine life.

Q20 | The pressure and blood gas data would be compatible with the problem being due to:

A. atrial septal defect
B. patent ductus arteriosus
C. patent ductus venosus
D. ventricular septal defect
E. aortic coarctation

Q21 | Considering the mechanisms that underlie baby L.'s inability to deliver adequate oxygen to his peripheral tissues, the situation might be resolved by administration of:

A. nitrates
B. prostaglandin E
C. a cyclo-oxygenase inhibitor
D. digitalis
E. a cardio-selective beta-adrenoreceptor agonist

The diagnosis is confirmed by echocardiography and a drug infusion is established. Baby L.'s symptoms begin to resolve within a few hours. By 4 days later, all cardiorespiratory parameters are normal and he is now mature enough no longer to require a humidicrib. Mother and infant progress normally, with no further problems.

Ms L. continues to avoid competitive athletics and becomes pregnant again within 15 months. This second pregnancy goes to term without incident.

MCQ ANSWERS AND FEEDBACK

1.C. Normal ovulation is always followed by a period of elevated body temperature, relative to the pre-ovulatory value, which persists until shortly before menstruation.

2.D. Elevated plasma progesterone has the effect of resetting the hypothalamic thermostat to a higher set-point. During pregnancy, this helps to optimize the thermal gradient between body and environment, facilitating removal of the additional metabolic heat generated by the rapidly growing fetoplacental unit.

3.B. As the corpus luteum is the source of the progesterone that elevates body temperature, the duration of the temperature shift represents the lifespan of the corpus luteum. This is normally around 14 days.

4.D. Progesterone release from the corpus luteum inhibits pituitary secretion of LH and follicle-stimulating hormone (FSH) and so prevents initiation of the next cycle of ovum development. Luteal progesterone and oestrogen both induce the endometrial proliferative changes that are necessary for implantation. These include growth of new blood vessels to provide a basis for the placental plate and synthesis of glycogen to provide metabolic substrates for the trophoblast.

5.E. Passage of the morula from oviduct into uterine cavity has occurred by around 4 days post fertilization, at which time the intrauterine fluid is nutritious enough to allow the morula to develop into a blastocyst. This process is complete by 7 days post fertilization. By then, sufficient endometrial glycogen has accumulated to allow local nutrition of the blastocyst over the initial week post implantation. However, continued luteal secretion of progesterone and oestrogen is needed for a further 7–10 days to stimulate enough endometrial blood vessel growth for establishment of a functional placenta.

6.C. The well-established link between strenuous athletic activity and disruption of the ovarian cycle in young women means that Ms L.'s sporting commitments are a very likely cause of her abnormal luteal phase. The problem seems to be one of insufficient time for implantation to become fully established: there is no evidence that ovulation is disrupted and measuring hormone levels is not going to provide any useful insight at this stage. Of course, if the patient continues to be infertile even after a period of reduced athletic activity, it may then be necessary to determine whether hormone levels are normal.

7.C. Plasma and urine hCG are detectable by radioassay as early as 1 day after implantation – that is, about 9 days after fertilization. However, the usual over-the-counter pregnancy testing kits, which rely on agglutination assay, are relatively insensitive and not reliable until about three weeks post fertilization. Plasma levels of oestrogens and progesterone do not start to rise above the non-pregnant range of values until about six weeks post fertilization and prolactin secretion rises even later.

8.B. You will recall that corpus luteal secretion during the ovarian cycle is stimulated by LH: this cannot occur once pregnancy has begun because pituitary release of LH is inhibited by the high plasma progesterone. So, in order to have continued hormone secretion from the corpus luteum, another source of gonadotrophic stimulation must be utilized.

9.A. Testosterone secretion from the fetal testes cannot be initiated unless hCG is present in the circulation. While hCG is also important for normal testicular descent, this process occurs only late in pregnancy.

10.A. In the presence of circulating progesterone, the mucus secreted by cervical endometrial glands is highly viscous. This forms a plug in the cervical opening and creates a physical seal to prevent intravaginal microorganisms entering the uterus.

11.C. Several hormones are needed to prepare the breast for lactation. Oestrogens stimulate formation of the duct system, progesterone stimulates maturation of the secretory glands, and prolactin and chorionic somatomammotrophin both act to induce production of the enzymes that will produce the milk.

12.C. Maternal cholesterol is converted to DHEA by the fetal adrenal and this DHEA is converted to oestrogens in the placenta. Over the first eight weeks of gestation these synthetic pathways are not effective because the fetal adrenal is immature and because the placenta is very small. During this time, all oestrogen production occurs in the corpus luteum.

13.D. Oestriol is the main oestrogen synthesized by the fetoplacental unit. Its production is proportional to both fetal metabolic integrity (which determines fetal conversion of cholesterol to DHEA) and to placental size (which determines rate of conversion of DHEA to oestriol). Oestradiol is the main oestrogen synthesized by the corpus luteum, but is produced only in small amounts by the fetoplacental unit. Oestradiol is therefore not a very sensitive indicator of fetoplacental growth. DHEA production is an index of fetal adrenal function, but it does not enter the maternal circulation, so it cannot easily be used as a marker of fetal growth. Progesterone and hCS provide indices of placental development, but do not provide information on fetal status.

14.E. The trigger appears to be a rise in the circulating ratio of oestrogen : progesterone. This stimulates induction of uterine oxytocin receptors and so allows the pre-existing plasma levels of oxytocin to initiate uterine contractions. There is some evidence that fetal cortisol may play a part in initiating labour, but maternal cortisol is not involved. Prostaglandins

synthesized in ruptured intrauterine membranes help maintain the labour process, but do not initiate it.

15.D. Prostaglandins are the only substances that act as myometrial excitants regardless of the stage of pregnancy. Those of the E series are generally preferred over the F series, because they produce fewer side-effects. Oxytocin stimulates myometrial contractility during normal labour because the high blood oestrogen levels induce uterine oxytocin receptors. However, since these receptors are almost absent until term, oxytocin is not an effective uterine stimulant at 37 weeks. Vasopressin contracts vascular smooth muscle cells but does not affect uterine motility. Activation of uterine beta-adrenoreceptors will cause relaxation of the pregnant uterus.

16.C. All neonates are relatively susceptible to cold. Because their surface area is high relative to their mass, they lose body heat rapidly. The surface area : mass ratio falls as development progresses, so premature infants are even less insulated than those at term. Immaturity of pulmonary surfactant secretion from alveolar type II cells is also a potential problem with premature births, although it is much more common with babies born prior to 35 weeks than at the age considered in this case. Both immune function and renal tubular mechanisms are immature in all neonates and do not develop fully for some weeks after birth.

17.A. Even though suction on the nipple is a major stimulus to milk ejection, mechanical stimulation alone is far less effective than actual suckling by the baby. Psychological stress can also inhibit the reflex pathway that causes oxytocin release. Prolactin secretion is also stimulated by suckling, and this is important for matching milk production to the baby's consumption. Here, however, we have a situation in which milk secretion is already occurring at a rate that engorges the breasts (so prolactin secretion must be adequate and the mammary ducts must exist) but ejection does not occur.

18.E. A pulse pressure of 60 mmHg is extremely high given the relatively high pulse rate. Diastolic pressure is normal in right ventricle but systolic value is above normal limits and both systolic and diastolic values are abnormally high in pulmonary artery and left atrium.

19.D. Neither respiratory function nor pulmonary blood flow can be deficient, since there is normal oxygenation of arterial plasma. The rapid ventilation and associated hypocapnia, with normal venous CO_2, indicate that the low systemic pH is due to metabolic acidosis. This could conceivably be caused by some peripheral metabolic defect but, as there is clear evidence of disturbed cardiac function, it is most likely that the problem is related to reduced systemic delivery of oxygenated blood, with resulting anaerobic metabolism and excess lactate production.

20.B. The ductus arteriosus normally closes during the 24 hours after birth. If this does not happen, a proportion of left heart ejection is shunted into the pulmonary artery, causing elevated right cardiac output and pulmonary arterial pressure. Such a situation is consistent with the present findings of high pulmonary blood pressure, high systolic right ventricular pressure (because of the increased afterload) and high left atrial pressure (because of the increased venous return). Because of the low peripheral resistance imposed by the ductal shunt, arterial pressure falls rapidly during diastole so pulse pressure is wide.

Functionally similar shunting of blood from left heart to pulmonary circulation could occur because of failure of the interventricular or interatrial septa to develop fully. However, the effects on regional pressures would be different to those of a ductal shunt. With an atrial septal defect, shunting of blood from left to right atrium would elevate right atrial pressure above its normal value. With an interventricular shunt, left stroke volume would be reduced and there would be compensatory peripheral vasoconstriction, leading to a narrow arterial pulse pressure. Elevation of aortic resistance by developmental coarctation would affect left heart pressures but would not alter those on the right side.

21.C. During fetal life, the ductus arteriosus is kept open by local production of prostaglandin E, which relaxes the ductus smooth muscle. Prostaglandin synthesis in this tissue is normally inhibited by increased Po_2, so the increased blood oxygenation that accompanies onset of air-breathing usually initiates ductus closure. The failure of closure that is seen in some premature infants and occasionally even after term delivery usually occurs because in these babies some prostaglandin synthesis continues. Inhibition of the remaining prostaglandin production with a cyclo-oxygenase antagonist such as indomethacin is therefore effective in stimulating closure. Nonetheless, in a subset of infants born with a patent ductus, this approach does not cause complete closure and in these cases surgical closure is necessary.

None of the other pharmacological approaches listed in this question would have any useful effect, since changes in cardiac function or peripheral resistance cannot alter the proportion of cardiac output that is lost through the ductal shunt.

CASE REVIEW

Irregularities of the menstrual cycle are often seen in women who undertake regular strenuous exercise such as competitive athletics. The underlying mechanisms are not clear, but a range of hormonal changes have been found suggesting that either or both of FSH and LH secretion may be depressed. The consequences vary from altered phase length, such as we saw in Ms L.'s shortened luteal phase, through to complete absence of ovulation and menstruation. In girls who begin strenuous activity before puberty, the onset of menstrual cycling (*menarche*) is often delayed.

Similar depression of hormonal cycling is seen in female ballet dancers and gymnasts and in girls who purposely starve themselves because of worries about their body image (*anorexia nervosa*). This distribution of occurrence suggests several possible triggers for disruption of hormone secretion, including low fat stores, emotional stress and adrenocortical hormone profiles.

We have seen from the present case that one consequence of this situation is temporary infertility, which is usually reversed within a few months of stopping training. There are, however, also long-term consequences of reduced gonadal steroid levels. One theoretical benefit is that the incidence of oestrogen-dependent tumours (uterine and breast) may be reduced. On the other hand, lack of oestrogens reduces bone mineralization, so these young women have an increased risk of stress fractures and potential osteoporosis.

It is not known what causes the syndrome of pre-eclampsia. The maternal cardiovascular and renal changes suggest that there might be some circulating vasoconstrictor substance, but no such factor has been convincingly isolated. There is some evidence that an autoimmune response leading to intravascular coagulation could be involved in at least some patients. The incidence of pre-eclampsia and of fetal growth retardation in general is more of a problem during a first pregnancy than later ones. In part, this is probably due to stress caused by psychological factors, but there is also some residual enlargement of the uterine blood vessels and uterine wall, which may provide better fetoplacental blood supply in later pregnancies. In Ms L.'s case, an additional factor retarding fetal growth may have been the fact that her endocrine regulation had not yet fully normalized following cessation of training.

Congenital abnormalities of the heart and associated great vessels are common, affecting around 1% of live births. About 40% of these cases involve ventricular septal defects, with atrial septal defects and patent ductus arteriosus being the next most common at 10% each. In many cases, the defects are not dramatic enough to cause obvious functional symptoms in childhood. However, where they induce additional cardiac work they are inevitably linked to increased long-term risk of heart failure. Defects like atrial fibrillation that have little effect on stroke volume in normal hearts may also have substantial effects when there is a pre-existing shunt.

KEY POINTS

- In young women, high levels of competitive physical activity in association with calorific restriction are often associated with reduced ovarian steroid secretion.
- This is due to reduced stimulation from the hypothalamo-pituitary axis.
- Consequences include infertility and reduced bone density.

- The success of implantation, pregnancy, labour and lactation are highly dependent on precisely timed interactions of a number of hormones.
- Understanding the roles of each hormone is essential in order to be able to interpret evidence of abnormal events.
- Congenital cardiac defects are common and should be repaired as early in life as is practicable.

ADDITIONAL READING

McGuire W, McEwan P & Fowlie PW (2004) Care in the early newborn period. *British Medical Journal* **329**: 1087–9.

Solomon CG & Seely EW (2004) Preeclampsia – searching for the cause. *New England Journal of Medicine* **350**: 641–2.

Warren MP & Perlroth NE (2001) The effects of intense exercise on the female reproductive system. *Journal of Endocrinology* **170**: 3–11.

Tight shoes and disturbed nights

CASE AND MCQS

Case introduction

A 60-year-old salesman, Mr J.S., attends your surgery complaining that over the past month or so he has felt breathless when going upstairs. He also notices that his shoes feel tight towards the end of a day. Occasionally he feels light-headed, but after sitting down soon feels better. He does not sleep well and often feels tired during the day.

Increasingly, he needs to pass urine several times at night and when he lies down he feels that his breathing becomes more laboured. He has found that this is relieved if he supports his head and neck with a couple of pillows. He has not taken much exercise for many years.

Examination reveals a thin man with pale skin and clammy hands. His arterial blood pressure is 170/110 mmHg; his pulse rate is 72–75 beats/min. Body temperature is normal and there are no signs of infection. Auscultation of his chest reveals light crackling noises associated with respiration (rales or crepitation) but no murmurs from cardiac valves can be detected.

The abdomen is slightly distended but the liver appears only marginally enlarged. Pitting oedema is detected with the fingers on the legs and ankles. A digital examination of the patient's rectum does not reveal evidence of an enlarged prostate gland.

Q1 In order to know more about cardiovascular status, you wish to measure central venous pressure. What is the routine clinical technique for this procedure?

A. an intravenous catheter and blood pressure transducer
B. visual inspection of peripheral superficial veins
C. measuring the height of the jugular venous column above the sternum
D. auscultation with a blood pressure manometer
E. palpation of the venous pulse

Mr S.'s central venous pressure, as measured by this technique, is 9 cm H_2O.

Q2 List the most important signs detected so far.

Q3 Can you draw any preliminary conclusions on the reasons for the symptoms? Do you think that they reflect problems that could be:

A. cardiac
B. respiratory
C. vascular
D. haematological
E. any of the above

Q4 Mr S.'s blood pressure has been measured as 170/110 mmHg. What are the normal levels of arterial blood pressure? Does pressure vary during the day? Is blood pressure likely to be affected by the environment?

You have noted that oedema is present in the legs and feet. Before taking the story further we need to look at some of the physiology that underlies the development of oedema.

Q5 Oedema is caused by:

A. subcutaneous proteoglycan deposition
B. increased interstitial fluid
C. enlarged superficial veins and capillaries
D. low haematocrit
E. both A and B above

Q6 In this patient, which observation is indicative of oedema in his legs and feet?

A. tight shoes
B. distended veins
C. appearance of superficial pits in skin when pressed
D. pale skin on the legs
E. all of the above

We need to think about the various physiological mechanisms involved in controlling the distribution of extracellular fluid across the wall between the interstitial space and the interior of a capillary. This is achieved through a balance of the Starling forces across the capillary wall: that is, the difference in hydrostatic pressure inside and outside of the capillary wall balanced against the osmotic pressures exerted by plasma protein and the normally small amounts of protein in the interstitial space.

Q7 Interstitial fluid:

A. has the same ionic composition as plasma
B. contains more potassium than plasma
C. contains more sodium than plasma
D. contains less sodium than plasma
E. contains less potassium than plasma

Q8 If the hydrostatic pressure inside the capillary increases:

A. fluid moves from the interstitial space into the capillary
B. fluid moves from the capillary into the interstitial space
C. fluid moves from the interstitial space into cells
D. fluid moves from cells into the interstitial space
E. there is no fluid movement provided that plasma oncotic pressure remains constant

Q9 Why does peripheral oedema occur more in the feet and lower legs than in other parts of the body?

A. capillary hydrostatic pressure is higher in the feet
B. plasma oncotic pressure is lower in the feet
C. arterial blood pressure is higher in the feet
D. peripheral resistance is lower in the feet
E. none of the above

Q10 Based on the symptoms displayed, oedema in the current case is likely to be caused by:

A. reduced peripheral resistance
B. reduced hepatic synthesis of plasma protein
C. increased capillary membrane permeability
D. increased peripheral venous pressure
E. a combination of A and B above

Q11 Under what circumstances could alterations in plasma protein become important? Think about the conditions that might cause this.

We now need to focus on the problems created by oedema, wherever it occurs. In this case there is evidence for oedema in the peripheral capillaries and in the lungs, as indicated by the patient's orthostatic dyspnoea.

Q12 Pulmonary oedema reduces gas transfer in the lungs primarily because it:

A. reduces respiratory rate and depth
B. increases the diffusion distance between alveolus and capillary
C. reduces alveolar exchange area
D. dilutes alveolar oxygen
E. washes surfactant away from the alveolar epithelial surface

You decide to have the following tests performed.
- Chest X ray: this shows some shadowing in the alveolar lung tissues, thus confirming the possibility of pulmonary oedema. The ventricles are enlarged. No other abnormalities are seen.
- Renal function: 24-hour urine collection and measurements of volume, urinary protein, urea, electrolytes and creatinine clearance show that all these variables are within normal limits.
- Blood: Red and white cell counts, haemoglobin, ESR (erythrocyte sedimentation rate), serum albumin and fasting glucose are all normal.

Q13 In identifying the underlying cause of oedema, the finding of a normal ESR is useful because it helps to exclude:

A. hepatic disease
B. infection
C. vascular disease
D. haematological disease
E. all of the above

It may be useful to summarize the most important symptoms we have seen so far:
- dyspnoea on gentle exercise
- signs of peripheral and pulmonary oedema
- raised jugular venous pressure
- high arterial blood pressure
- orthopnoea
- nocturnal diuresis
- but no signs of major cardiac valve problems.

What preliminary conclusions can you reach?

Q14 Mr S. is *not* likely to be suffering from:

A. aortic stenosis
B. kidney disease
C. cardiac myopathy
D. diabetes insipidus
E. any of the above

We now need to look at possible reasons for the raised capillary pressures in the pulmonary and systemic circulations – remember the oedema. Mr S. is hypertensive and it is therefore useful to consider the ways in which a high arterial blood pressure might affect the heart and circulation.

Q15 In the presence of high arterial blood pressure:

A. end-systolic left ventricular volume is increased
B. end-systolic left ventricular volume is decreased
C. end-diastolic left ventricular volume is decreased
D. systolic ejection fraction is increased
E. none of the above

Initially, the effect of an increased afterload is to increase the force of contraction of the ventricles (Starling's law), but only if the muscle is not stretched too far (look up the relation between diastolic pressure and stroke volume). With moderate elevation of end-diastolic volume stroke volume increases, but it then falls if the fibres are stretched beyond the optimal length of muscle fibre for producing active tension. It should be noted that the pericardium restricts the expansion of the heart and so helps to prevent this passive overstretching.

The reduced outflow from both ventricles will result in an increase in left and right atrial pressures and if these rise sufficiently, there will be elevation of pulmonary and systemic capillary hydrostatic pressures, leading to oedema. So, hypertension alone may be part of the explanation for Mr S.'s symptoms.

Since there are several established pharmacological measures that will reduce the blood pressure effectively and selectively, you decide to use this approach first. Beta-blockers (beta-adrenoreceptor antagonists) reduce the vascular and cardiac effects of circulating catecholamines; diuretic agents will reduce the overall blood volume; selective calcium-channel blockers will reduce the contraction of vascular smooth muscle as will angiotensin-converting enzyme (ACE) inhibitors. All will reduce arterial blood pressure in the appropriate doses.

Q16 ACE inhibitors:

A. reduce the production of renin
B. reduce the production of angiotensin II
C. reduce the production of angiotensin I
D. reduce the production of angiotensinogen
E. none of the above

Q17   **ACE inhibitors lower blood pressure by:**

A.   increasing renal sodium excretion
B.   reducing the plasma concentration of aldosterone
C.   increasing water excretion
D.   causing vasodilation
E.   all of the above

You send Mr S. away with a prescription for a diuretic. But you have in mind that raised arterial blood pressure is unlikely to be the sole cause of the relatively severe oedema seen in this case and that other factors may be operating.

One month later, it is clear that this prescription is not working effectively. When you now re-examine him his blood pressure is normalized (125/85 mmHg) but the major symptoms remain. The next stage is to look at the function of the heart since the remaining symptoms are likely to involve problems within the 'pump' itself. You send Mr S. for further tests at the hospital.

It may be useful to list the various investigations that can be carried out and the specific information that each will provide. Some information is shown below, but you may be able to think of additional factors:

Non-invasive tests

• Electrocardiogram – indicates arrhythmias, infarction, ischaemia, left or right ventricular hypertrophy
• Chest X-ray – indicates size of chambers of the heart, especially ventricles
• Echocardiogram – assesses action of valves and enables identification of possible blockage of the valves or other dysfunction
• Doppler echocardiography – visualizes detail of cardiac chambers, enables calculation of ejection fraction
• Exercise stress testing – tests ability of heart to respond to demands for increased oxygen in active skeletal muscles in a controlled way, identifies ischaemic heart disease.

Invasive tests

• Coronary angiography – identifies partial or full blockage of coronary arteries which will reduce the supply of blood to the active cardiac muscle
• Radionuclide tests – infusions of specific radiolabelled agents enable specific aspects of ventricular physiology and function to be evaluated.

The details of these tests are available in standard cardiology texts.

Back to this case. You ask for a 12-channel ECG to be performed. A portion of the record obtained is shown in Fig. 6.1.

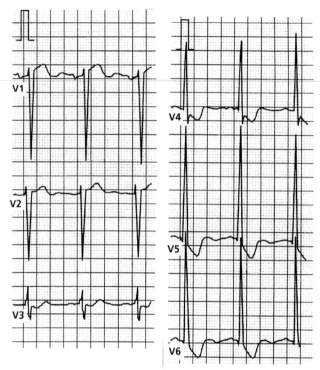

Fig. 6.1 Chest lead ECGs (V1–V6) recorded from J.S.

Q18   **This ECG indicates:**

A.   ventricular hypertrophy
B.   complete heart block
C.   1:2 heart block
D.   ventricular hypertrophy and complete heart block
E.   a normal heart

Chest X-ray shows enlarged left and right ventricles. A cardiac echocardiogram is also performed. This indicates that all cardiac valves are operating normally and that the ejection fraction is 30%.

Q19   **What is the normal ejection fraction?**

A.   40%
B   60%
C.   80%
D.   100%
E.   none of the above

An exercise stress test indicates a significantly reduced exercise tolerance, clear evidence of coronary bed ischaemia. It is not judged necessary to perform an angiographic study of the coronary arteries at this stage.

It is concluded that while the echocardiogram indicates no valve problems, Mr S. is suffering from a failure of his cardiac muscle to contract effectively. His inability to pump the blood through the chambers effectively has resulted in enlargement of the atria and ventricles on both sides: this has in turn led to raised atrial and venous pressures with consequent pulmonary and peripheral venous congestion.

Further treatment should be aimed at reducing the workload of the heart and strengthening the vigour of contraction of the cardiac muscle. Additional investigations will be needed to identify further the reasons for the cardiac muscle dysfunction. These could include metabolic dysfunction, viral myocarditis or an infiltrative disease. Further examination could determine if a previous 'silent' heart attack had resulted in damage to part of the myocardium which had not been detected by electrocardiography. Possible investigations for this purpose would include coronary angiography and/or radionuclide imaging studies.

Other studies would be aimed at showing whether the problem lies in the systolic action of the heart or in some aspect of diastolic function, such as stiffening of the ventricle or the pericardium that limits ventricular filling. For us, further detailed examination at this stage is not helpful as we have identified the main physiological factors that underlie the symptoms.

MCQ ANSWERS AND FEEDBACK

1.C. Jugular venous pressure is the standard index of central venous pressure. It is measured non-invasively with the patient lying on a bed and the head supported on pillow. The height above the sternal angle at which the internal jugular vein collapses marks central venous pressure. Normally, jugular venous pressure (JVP) is approximately 6 cmH$_2$O.

2. Dyspnoea on slight exercise; high arterial blood pressure; some signs of peripheral and pulmonary oedema; raised JVP; orthopnoea; nocturnal diuresis; no signs of major cardiac valve problems.

3.E. At this preliminary stage, none could be sensibly excluded.

4. Normal arterial blood pressure is usually stated to be 120/80 mmHg. However, it varies greatly during the day with activity and mood and is particularly low during sleep. Generally a resting systolic pressure over 140 mmHg or a diastolic pressure over 90 mmHg is now regarded as being one that requires attention in some way, with selective elevation of systolic pressure being especially common in elderly people. In many individuals the fact of taking their blood pressure is sufficient to raise it significantly (the 'white coat' effect). How would you ensure that this error was minimized when measuring a patient's blood pressure?

5.B. By definition, oedema is an increase in interstitial fluid volume.

6.C. 'Pitting' of the skin in the lower limbs and feet is diagnostic. Tight shoes, venous distension and pallor could all have several explanations.

7.A. Interstitial fluid is an ultra-filtrate of plasma; plasma protein is the only constituent that cannot pass across the capillary wall. Hence the ionic compositions of the two compartments are identical.

8.B. The plasma protein exerts an oncotic (= colloid osmotic) pressure tending to draw fluid back into the capillary, which is substantially larger than the pressure exerted by the small amount of free protein in the interstitial space. If intracapillary pressure becomes greater than interstitial pressure and oncotic pressures remain the same, water movement must be from plasma to interstitium. Fluid movement between these compartments has no effect on intracellular fluid unless the composition of the interstitial fluid changes.

9.A. When standing, capillary pressure in the legs and feet is higher than in the upper limbs, because there is a continuous column of blood between the heart and the feet. Thus, in the feet, there is a gravitational pressure of around 150 cmH$_2$O in the capillaries on top of the normal hydrostatic pressure of around 40 mmHg.

You can estimate the gravitational effect on intracapillary pressure in mmHg using the fact that the density of mercury is 13.6 times that of water. The gravitational force means that arterial pressure is also higher in the feet than at heart level in a standing person but, since there can be no water movement across the arterial wall, it is the intracapillary pressure that is important in determining whether oedema occurs.

10.D. You know that central venous pressure is elevated and this will be reflected in a rise in peripheral venous and capillary pressure. The other alternatives could also lead to oedema but there is no evidence that they are likely to be involved in this patient. In particular, his high blood pressure indicates that his peripheral resistance is if anything elevated above normal.

11. Reduced plasma protein concentration and reduced oncotic pressure can occur during severe famine and starvation or as a result of liver or kidney disease. Also, a small amount of protein does leak out of the circulation and is recycled back into the venous system via the lymphatics. Widespread damage to the lymphatics will impair this recycling.

12.B. Any increase in the diffusion distance between the alveoli and plasma has a dramatic effect on transfer of respiratory gases, especially oxygen from alveoli to plasma. If pulmonary oedema is sufficient to cause movement of fluid into the alveoli this will further impair respiratory efficiency by diluting surfactant and making it harder to inflate the lungs. The effects of oedema on gas transfer are the same at the peripheral capillary/tissue interface and can profoundly affect the unloading and uploading of gases, especially oxygen, at the tissue level.

13.B. Elevated erythrocyte sedimentation rate is useful as a non-specific indicator of infection.

14.E. None of the alternatives is compatible with the combination of symptoms shown by this patient. Aortic stenosis and cardiac myopathy would be associated with reduced blood pressure and his normal renal function data exclude kidney disease or diabetes insipidus.

15.A. The high arterial blood pressure represents an additional load against which the heart has to eject blood (= increased afterload) and so it has to generate higher intra-ventricular pressures to eject the same amount of blood and/

or eject less blood. Since venous return continues at the same rate as before, reduced ventricular emptying (stroke volume) will increase the end-diastolic volume of the heart. Therefore, ejection fraction (end-systolic volume/end-diastolic volume) will also fall.

16.B. Inhibition of angiotensin-converting enzyme (ACE) will reduce the production of angiotensin II from angiotensin I, which is in turn derived by the action of renin on the plasma alpha-globulin, angiotensinogen. Renin comes from the juxtaglomerular cells of the renal afferent arteriole.

17.E. Angiotensin II increases arterial blood pressure via vasoconstriction and the ACE inhibitor will induce a fall though this mechanism. Angiotensin II also stimulates sodium reabsorption in the renal tubule; chloride and water follow passively. It also stimulates aldosterone secretion from the adrenal cortex which will in turn affect sodium reabsorption in the kidney and secretion of antidiuretic hormone from the posterior pituitary gland. Inhibition of all of these actions will tend to reduce arterial blood pressure and increase urine flow.

18.A. With a normal amount of ventricular muscle tissue, the R wave is never greater than 2.5 mV in any lead. The R waves in this recording of up to 3 mV or more indicate a substantial degree of ventricular hypertrophy. Each QRS complex is preceded by a P wave and the frequency of ventricular activation is normal at around 70 beats/min (remember that each square on the ECG record represents 200 ms), so every atrial impulse is reaching the ventricle – that is, there is no atrioventricular block.

19.B. Typically, the end-diastolic ventricular volume is around 120 ml and stroke volume is around 70 ml.

CASE REVIEW

This case study has discussed three possible malfunctions of physiological mechanisms that can underlie heart failure. These are not the only examples of disturbed physiology that could have been described. Essentially, cardiac failure is present when the output of the left ventricle fails to match the metabolic demands of the body or does so only when the cardiac filling pressure is high. Think about the factors that affect flow of blood through the heart and consider how cardiac failure might result from other physiological disturbances.

Many patients suffering from heart failure remain asymptomatic for long periods, either because the impairment is mild or because the cardiac dysfunction is balanced by compensatory mechanisms elsewhere. Such patients are regarded as being adequately 'compensated'. Often the clinical features

of failure only appear as a result of precipitating factors that increase cardiac workload and tip the balance into their being 'decompensated'.

The natural physiological compensating mechanisms include Starling's law, progressive hypertrophy of the cardiac muscle and neurohormonal activation. The latter includes the actions of the adrenergic nervous system, renin–angiotensin system, antidiuretic hormone (ADH, vasopressin) and atrial natriuretic peptide (ANP). Each or all can operate to have positive and negative effects under different circumstances.

These compensating processes can be disturbed by other precipitating factors including alterations in circulating blood volume (causing increased preload), increased blood pressure (causing increased afterload), impaired contractility (causing reduced stroke volume) and increased metabolic demand (causing reduced peripheral resistance). So, heart failure can be the result of altered physiology in several different systems. But the contribution of each can be isolated and the results used to form the basis of a rational scientific approach to the treatment of symptoms.

It may be useful if you were to make up a flow diagram that summarizes the factors involved during cardiac failure in the transition between compensation and decompensation.

In relation to oedema, we have been explaining it in relation to current and well-established hypotheses. Like most areas of physiology these do evolve and the two short papers in the reading list below illustrate that new ideas, based on new evidence, on how the processes work arise constantly.

Dyspnoea is one of the early symptoms of heart failure, although of course there can be causes of dyspnoea other than heart failure and these need to be excluded. In heart failure, dyspnoea can result from several processes and the relative contributions of these may vary at different phases:

1. Inability to supply adequate cardiac output for the muscular metabolic demands being imposed will lead to hypercapnia.
2. Pulmonary venous congestion will result in transudation of plasma into the pulmonary interstitium. As well as reducing gas exchange directly, this would reduce pulmonary compliance and elevate airways resistance as a result of the compressing the airways and alveoli.

These changes would both increase the work of breathing since the patient would need to generate a greater negative intrathoracic pressure to move the same amount of air.

3. Finally, pulmonary oedema could stimulate juxtacapillary receptors (J-receptors) and result in reflex production of rapid, shallow breathing.

Dyspnoea sometimes occurs in patients without overt pulmonary oedema, probably because there is failure of the cardiac muscle to generate an adequate blood flow to the respiratory muscles. Inevitably, dyspnoea is likely to become progressively greater as the cardiac failure (pumping action) becomes more severe: eventually, even gentle walking becomes difficult.

KEY POINTS

- Cardiac failure represents a mismatch between cardiac output and the metabolic demands of the body.
- It may be due to a primary defect in the myocardium or be secondary to a mismatch between the functional limits of the heart and the volume it is required to pump.
- Regardless of the cause, cardiac failure is characterized by dyspnoea and by peripheral oedema.
- Effective treatment depends on logical analysis of the potential sites of malfunction of the heart.

ADDITIONAL READING

Levick JR (2002) *An Introduction to Cardiovascular Physiology*, 4th edition. Arnold, London.

Levick JS (2004) Revision of the Starling principle: new views of tissue balance. *Journal of Physiology, London* 557: 704.

Lilly LR (ed.) (1998) *Pathophysiology of Heart Disease*, 2nd edition. Williams & Wilkins, Baltimore.

Michel CC (2004) Fluid exchange in the microcirculation. *Journal of Physiology, London* 557: 701–2.

Patterson D & Treasure T (eds) (1995) *Disorders of the Cardiovascular System*. Arnold, London.

Sore throat and bloating

CASE AND MCQS

Case introduction

J.K., a 22-year-old man, normal weight 72 kg (159 lb), presents to the doctor's surgery with a history that over the last 4 days he had developed swelling of his legs, hands and face. Approximately a week before this started he had a sore throat which resolved without treatment. He has noticed that he has been passing less urine and drinking more fluid. He says that his urine is clear and of normal colour.

He has had two similar episodes in the past, which had resolved with treatment, both occurring after a sore throat. The first was at the age of 17, the second when he was 19 years of age.

On examination, the patient appears puffy and has swelling of his legs with pitting oedema up to his mid-thighs. His hands are swollen.

Blood pressure is 115/75 mmHg; pulse rate is 65 beats/min. Jugular venous pressure is not elevated. There is a suggestion of shifting dullness in the abdominal cavity.

Urine analysis is performed, samples are taken for plasma biochemistry and haematology and a 24-hour urine collection is commenced. The patient's file and records of the previous admissions are requested.

 Q1 Which of the following is the most likely cause of Mr K.'s gross oedema? (Do not be concerned if you cannot answer this question at this stage)

A. cardiac failure
B. liver disease
C. nephrotic syndrome
D. acute glomerulonephritis
E. lymphoedema

Q2 Which of the following is most likely to be found in Mr K.'s urine?

A. red cells and red cell casts
B. protein
C. red cells, red cell casts and protein
D. no abnormality
E. protein and protein casts

Mr K.'s plasma biochemistry before this episode gave the following normal results:

Sodium	141 mmol/l
Potassium	4.4 mmol/l
Creatinine	0.08 mmol/l
Albumin	41 g/l

Q3 Which of the profiles below is the most likely result for his plasma biochemistry at presentation?

	Na$^+$ (mmol/l)	K$^+$ (mmol/l)	Creatinine (mmol/l)	Albumin (g/l)
A	138	4.3	0.08	34
B	125	3.8	0.12	22
C	138	3.8	0.07	22
D	139	4.5	0.12	22
E	145	5.3	0.07	22

Q4 Assuming that the values for glomerular filtration rate (GFR), haematocrit and haemoglobin before this episode were normal, which of the profiles below is most likely to be found at presentation?

	GFR (ml/min)	Haematocrit (%)	Haemoglobin (g/dl)
A	110	42	15.5
B	120	44	16.0
C	120	38	14.1
D	90	38	14.1
E	70	38	14.1

Normal values for J.K.: GFR 110 ml/min; haematocrit 42%; haemoglobin 15.5 g/dl.

Q5 From the results of the clinical examination, how much water do you think Mr K. has retained?

A. 1 litre
B. 3 litres
C. 5 litres
D. 15 litres
E. 25 litres

The results of the investigations are returned. The urine shows protein +++ and protein casts, with no red cells. Blood analysis shows:

Sodium	138 mmol/l
Potassium	3.8 mmol/l
Creatinine	0.07 mmol/l
Urea	3.8 mmol/l
Albumin	21 g/l
Total protein	55 g/l
Haematocrit	45%
Haemoglobin	16.2 g/dl

Mr K.'s GFR is 120 ml/min, 24-hour urine protein is 8 g/day. His weight is now 85 kg (187 lb), having been 72 kg (159 lb) prior to this episode.

These data confirm that protein is being excreted in the urine, leading to a low plasma albumin, with retention of sodium and water in the body and gross oedema. This confirms a diagnosis of nephrotic syndrome.

To understand the nephrotic syndrome it is important to understand how protein is normally handled by the kidney and the following questions relate to the control of glomerular filtration and protein handling.

Q6 Which of the following statements related to glomerular filtration is not correct?

A. efferent arteriole constriction increases GFR
B. afferent arteriole constriction increases GFR
C. a high protein oncotic pressure reduces GFR
D. the filtration fraction in humans is about 20%
E. glomerular capillary hydrostatic pressure is about 50 mmHg

Q7 Which of the following statements related to glomerular filtration and proteinuria is not correct?

A. plasma solutes with a molecular weight <8000 have a filtration coefficient close to one
B. the filtration coefficient for albumin in a normal person is <0.001
C. about 7 g albumin is filtered each day
D. proteins lost into the urine as a result of defective tubular function are predominantly basic (anionic)
E. basic (anionic) proteins are filtered by the glomerulus more than cationic proteins of the same molecular weight

Q8 Which of the following statements is correct for a normal individual?

A. albumin is not filtered
B. albumin is filtered and is not reabsorbed
C. urinary loss of albumin is around 110 mg/day
D. albumin is filtered and is destroyed by the proximal tubule cells
E. albumin is secreted by the proximal tubule cells

Q9 In a person who has retained 13 kg of fluid and whose plasma albumin has fallen from 42 to 21 g/l (i.e. a fall of 50%), which of the following statements is most likely to be true?

A. total body albumin has increased
B. total body albumin has not changed
C. total body albumin has decreased by about 60%
D. total body albumin has decreased by about 50%
E. total body albumin has decreased by about 40%

In the present case, assessment of Mr K's weight gain indicates that he has retained 13 litres of fluid. As a consequence, he has become oedematous. This means that fluid has been re-distributed from the plasma compartment of the interstitial space, and salt and water has been retained by the kidney and has also moved into the interstitial space.

The following questions are related to the forces that control the distribution between plasma and the interstitial compartment.

Figure 7.1 shows the forces that control the movement of fluid at the arterial and venous ends of a tissue capillary. The forces are:
• Capillary hydrostatic pressure (CHP)
• Capillary oncotic pressure (COP)
• Tissue oncotic pressure (TOP)
• Tissue hydrostatic pressure (THP)
• Net force out at arterial end (Net)
• Net force in at venous end (Net).

Q10 Complete Fig. 7.1 by indicating the approximate values next to each of these forces and show the direction of force by adding an arrowhead symbol on each line.

Q11 Which of the following is *least* likely to cause accumulation of fluid in the interstitium?

A. elevation of arterial blood pressure, e.g. essential hypertension
B. low plasma albumin
C. increased capillary permeability to albumin
D. increased venous pressure, e.g. heart failure
E. lymphatic obstruction

To return to our current patient – the fluid retention is causing discomfort and some problems. Consider what you could do to reduce the fluid accumulation.

Q12 Which of the following therapies would be your first choice at this stage in this patient?

A. albumin infusion
B. high-dose thiazide diuretic
C. low-dose furosemide
D. high-dose furosemide
E. both A and D

Q13 What are the potential dangers of successful diuresis achieved with a diuretic in a person with the nephrotic syndrome?

A. hyperkalaemia
B. hypokalaemia
C. increased haematocrit
D. both A and C
E. both B and C

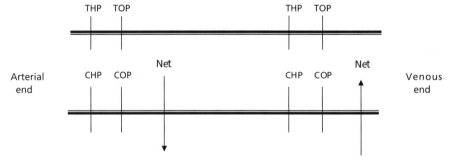

Fig. 7.1 Incomplete diagram of the forces that control the movement of fluid at the arterial and venous ends of a tissue capillary.

Mr K. informs you that on the two previous occasions he had been treated with prednisolone 60 mg as a once-daily dose and this had caused a diuresis and reversal of his disease. Inspection of his past record indicates that on his first admission he had been unwell for about 10 days before presentation. He had had a renal biopsy that showed minor changes in the glomeruli.

His biochemistry on that admission was:

Sodium	141 mmol/l
Potassium	3.8 mmol/l
Creatinine	0.09 mmol/l
Urea	4.4 mmol/l
Albumin	16 g/l
Total protein	45 g/l
Globulin	29 g/l
Cholesterol	7.5 mmol/l
Haemoglobin	17 g/dl
Haematocrit	48%

His GFR was 100 ml/min, his blood pressure had fallen to 90/60 mmHg and his 24-hour urine protein excretion was 5 g/day.

He had been given furosemide 40 mg i.v. and on the next day 100 mg i.v., with little effect on either occasion. On day 15 after his initial problem began he was given prednisolone 60 mg.

In the next 48 hours he had a diuresis of 22 litres and lost 18 kg (40 lb) in weight. His albumin rose over 48 hours from 16 to 32 g/l and his blood pressure rose to 115/75 mmHg.

There was an initial fall in plasma potassium to 3.4 mmol/l, but 72 hours after starting therapy his blood values were:

Sodium	140 mmol/l
Potassium	3.9 mmol/l
Creatinine	0.07 mmol/l
Urea	2.4 mmol/l

Albumin	32 g/l
Total protein	71 g/l
Haemoglobin	15.8 g/dl
Haematocrit	42%

The steroid therapy was gradually stopped and the proteinuria did not return.

The second episode, when he was 19, was similar to the present one and had also been reversed with steroid therapy. On that occasion, the 24-hour protein excretion after remission was <300 mg/day.

Q14 The filtration barrier to proteins in the glomerulus involves:

A. axial streaming
B. the fenestrae of the capillary
C. the slit diaphragm
D. both A and B
E. all of A, B and C

Q15 In a person with nephrotic syndrome, which one of the following statements is *not* correct?

A. the light microscopy of the glomerulus may be relatively normal on biopsy
B. the glomerulus may exhibit membranous nephritis
C. the nephrotic syndrome may be due to tubular disease
D. the urine may contain red cells
E. measured blood volume may be normal

The renal biopsy was relatively normal by light microscopy, but important abnormalities were seen on electron microscopy.

There was an excellent response to steroid therapy with no recurrence of problems over the next six months.

MCQ ANSWERS AND FEEDBACK

1.C. Acute glomerulonephritis rarely causes gross oedema. All of the others can cause gross oedema but if it were due to cardiac failure the JVP would be elevated. If it were due to liver disease, other signs of liver disease would be expected. Lymphoedema, due to obstruction of lymph flow, is usually a chronic and not an acute problem. The most likely cause of sudden gross oedema is protein loss by the kidney leading to a low plasma albumin, fluid retention and gross oedema. This complex of signs is called the nephrotic syndrome. The characteristics of nephrotic syndrome are:
- Glomerular damage
- Increased albumin and protein filtration exceeding reabsorptive capacity of tubule

- Proteinuria
- Low serum albumin
- Reduced plasma volume
- Fluid retention
- Gross oedema
- Hyperlipidaemia.

2.E. Severe nephrotic syndrome of this nature will probably be associated only with protein and protein casts in the urine.

3.C. To have this degree of oedema, albumin would need to be below 25 g/l. Creatinine would not be expected to be elevated early in the course of the nephrotic syndrome and, in actual fact, may be reduced. Sodium concentration would usually be in the normal range. Potassium would tend to be lower due to increased aldosterone levels following the acute volume depletion.

4.B. Early in the nephrotic syndrome, GFR tends to rise due to the effect of a low plasma albumin on the glomerular filtration forces. There is a functional reduction in blood volume and thus both haematocrit and haemoglobin will tend to be higher. Thus B is the most likely answer, although A is also a (less likely) possibility.

5.D. If pitting oedema is present at the ankles this means that 1 or 2 litres of fluid have been retained. Pitting oedema up to the thighs, with the possibility of some ascites, would indicate that 10–15 litres have been retained. You could calculate this by estimating the volume needed to increase the diameter of a cylinder by 1 cm in each leg.

6.B. The hydrostatic pressure in the glomerular capillaries is about 55 mmHg and this favours filtration (Fig. 7.2). It is opposed by the protein oncotic pressure and thus high protein oncotic pressure reduces GFR while a low protein oncotic pressure (low albumin) increases GFR. Efferent arteriole constriction causes an increase in glomerular pressure and this increases GFR. Afferent arteriole constriction causes a reduction in blood flow and a reduction in glomerular hydrostatic pressure, and thus a fall in GFR. Usually about 20% of plasma is filtered, i.e. a filtration faction of 20%. In contrast to tissue capillaries there is little or no drop in pressure between the arterial and venous end.

7.E. The glomerular capillaries are very permeable and substances smaller than 8000 Da (= molecular weight of 8000) are filtered in proportion to water. That is a filtration coefficient of 1.0. The barrier to large molecules depends on the size and the charge. The filtration barrier has a negative charge and thus cationic proteins of the same size are filtered more than anionic proteins. However, in plasma, the smaller proteins are anionic and thus anionic (basic) proteins appear in the urine in tubular disease. Albumin, even though it has a molecular weight of 70 000, is filtered to a small extent (filtration coefficient of about 0.001). This means that 7 g of protein is filtered each day.

8.D. Albumin is filtered to a small extent in a normal person, and the albumin filtered is taken up by endocytosis in the proximal tubule cells and is broken down to amino acids which go back into the bloodstream. The urine is close to albumin-free (<30 mg/day).

9.E. Albumin has been lost and the plasma albumin has fallen by 50%. However, the total body albumin will not be decreased as much because the interstitial fluid contains some albumin, though at a lower concentration than in plasma.

10. The values given in Fig. 7.3 are representative values from muscle capillaries, but values can vary in different tissues and under different degrees of activities. Textbooks frequently show the tissue oncotic pressure as zero but there is protein, including albumin, in the interstitial space. The albumin concentration is between 10 and 20% of that in plasma. In contrast to glomerular capillaries, less than 2% of the fluid goes into the interstitium and most re-enters the capillary. What is not returned re-enters the circulation via the lymphatics. The drop in hydrostatic pressure along the capillary is what alters the balance of forces.

11.A. If there were elevation of hydrostatic pressure at the arterial end of the capillary, A would be correct. However, in-

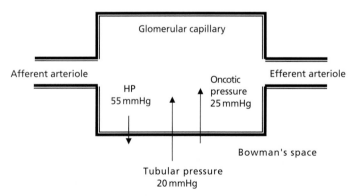

Fig. 7.2 The glomerular capillaries form a network and there is little pressure drop between the arterial and venous ends. The pressures are higher in this network than in the tissue capillaries as it is in the arterial circulation. Filtration forces and filtration rate are high at the start of the network but as water is lost with the filtrate the protein concentration and thus the oncotic pressure rises and filtration is completed before the end of the capillary network. The hydrostatic pressure (HP) in the glomerular capillary depends on the systemic blood pressure and the tone (degree of constriction) of the afferent and efferent arterioles.

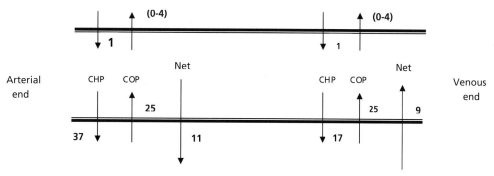

Fig. 7.3 Completed diagram of the forces that control the movement of fluid at the arterial and venous ends of the tissue capillary.

creased arterial pressure, as in essential hypertension, results from the constriction of the precapillary arteriole. Thus hydrostatic pressure is not elevated in the capillary even though it is elevated in the arterial system. All of the other situations can cause oedema.

12.C. Albumin infusion would work acutely, but the albumin is filtered and lost in the urine and the response is short lived. Thiazide diuretics work on the distal part of the nephron where relatively little fluid is absorbed, particularly in a volume-depleted state. Thus we need to use a diuretic that works on the loop of Henle (such as furosemide). We start with a low dose as rapid diuresis can cause acute problems (see Question 13).

13.E. A rapid diuresis would probably cause hypokalaemia as there is already increased aldosterone. It would also cause acute loss of fluid from the vascular compartment which would be replenished only slowly from the interstitial compartment. Thus the haematocrit would increase and may cause problems due to thrombosis.

14.C. The barrier to filtration of proteins is complex. The axial streaming of protein is important, the fenestrae of the capillaries are important, as also is the slit diaphragm. These hold up proteins at different sites, depending on the size.

15.C. While about 7 g/day of albumin is filtered, this is not sufficient to cause the nephrotic syndrome even if none is reabsorbed by the tubules. Patients with nephrotic syndrome can have a relatively normal renal biopsy or membranous glomerulonephritis and have proteinuria as the principal defect. It can also occur with proliferative glomerulonephritis when there are red cells in the urine as well as protein. Blood volume may be restored close to normal when it is compensated. When it is measured, blood volume may be within the normal range though mechanistically it is initially reduced.

CASE REVIEW

This is the third episode of severe oedema occurring after an upper respiratory tract infection. J.K. almost certainly has nephrotic syndrome, as this is a major cause of sudden development of fluid retention and oedema. He probably has a large amount of protein in his urine and there would be protein casts.

After a streptococcal sore throat, renal disease may develop as acute post-streptococcal glomerulonephritis, but it is unusual for this to develop into the nephrotic syndrome and is unlikely to be recurrent. However, viral infections in some people can trigger an immune process that causes increased glomerular capillary permeability and proteinuria. If this is sufficiently severe it will lead to the nephrotic syndrome. As J.K. is grossly oedematous, his plasma albumin will be below 30. His sodium and potassium would probably be normal.

The factors involved in the control of glomerular filtration are as follows:
• Glomerular capillary very permeable
• Molecular weight <8000; filtration coefficient = 1
• Filtration forces controlled by arteriolar tone
• Increased afferent tone – decreases pressure, flow and filtration
• Increased efferent tone – increases pressure and filtration
• Filtration fraction ≈ 20%
• Individual nephron control
• Tubuloglomerular feedback.

Early in the nephrotic syndrome GFR may be increased and renal functional deterioration would occur only if the patient is severely hypotensive. With an increase in GFR, haematocrit and haemoglobin would also be slightly increased due to a reduction in circulating plasma volume. GFR rises because of the fall in plasma albumin altering the forces at the glomerulus capillary. The hydrostatic pressure in the glomerulus will be increased by constriction of the efferent arteriole which will cause a rise in GFR and an increase in filtration fraction from its usual value of about 20%.

The glomerular membrane is very permeable and substances with a molecular weight <8000 pass through at the same concentration as in plasma. Even molecules as large as albumin can pass through and the filtration coefficient for albumin is about 0.001. This, however, means that about 7 g of albumin is filtered each day and this albumin is taken up by the proximal tubule by endocytosis and broken down in tubule cells to amino acids. In a healthy person, most of the albumin is removed so that less than 30 mg/day are excreted in the urine.

The glomerular membranes bear anionic charges so, in addition to size, the charge of a protein determines its filtration. Anionic proteins of the same size are filtered less than cationic proteins. However, plasma contains a number of anionic proteins with a molecular weight less than albumin and when there is tubular damage anionic proteins are found in the urine.

J.K. has had damage to his glomerular capillaries and is filtering a large amount of albumin. The amount filtered is much greater than that excreted in the urine because the proximal tubule reabsorbs proteins and breaks them down to amino acids. Initially, there may have been 20–40 g of albumin/day in the urine, but the fall in plasma concentration reduces the amount filtered (GFR × plasma concentration × filtration coefficient). The loss of albumin in the urine and the large destruction by the proximal tubule exceeds the liver's ability to synthesize albumin, so plasma albumin falls. This fall alters the filtration forces in the glomerulus and tissue capillaries, leading to an initial increase in GFR and movement of fluid into the tissues.

The reduction in circulating blood volume causes elevation of haematocrit and haemoglobin, but also activates hormonal systems, causing aldosterone secretion and salt and water retention. The fluid retention is an attempt to restore plasma volume, but instead it continues to be extravasated into the tissues because of the low oncotic pressure. When a person has pitting oedema up to mid-thighs, generalized oedema and fluid in the abdomen, at least 15 litres of fluid has accumulated (calculate how much fluid is needed to increase the diameter of the cylinder 90 cm long, diameter 15 cm, by 2 cm).

In the case of J.K., the plasma concentration of albumin has fallen by 50%, but the fall in total body albumin is less, as the retained interstitial fluid of 15 litres or more will contain some albumin. A similar sequence of events will occur with low plasma albumin, no matter what the cause. It may result from impaired protein synthesis due to liver disease or poor synthesis due to protein malnutrition. In those circumstances, however, the onset is gradual. By contrast, the onset is often very rapid when protein loss is via the urine. Figure 7.4 summarizes the events that lead to salt and water retention and oedema in the presence of low plasma albumin.

It is possible to induce diuresis by infusing albumin and, if a patient is severely hypotensive, this may be needed. However, the infused albumin is rapidly lost in the urine so the effect is brief. The usual procedure if there is gross oedema would be to give a low dose of furosemide. If, however, a large diuresis resulted, this could cause severe hypokalaemia as there is a large amount of aldosterone present and it would also remove fluid from the circulating plasma, leading to a rise in haematocrit and also a fall in blood pressure. Thus, caution is needed.

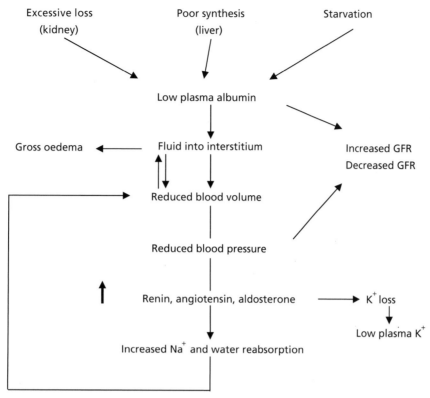

Fig. 7.4 Causes of salt and water retention in the presence of low plasma albumin.

KEY POINTS

- The forces controlling glomerular filtration are similar to the Starling's forces at the tissue capillary, but of a different magnitude.
- Glomerular capillaries are more permeable than tissue capillaries.
- Twenty per cent of the renal plasma flow is filtered.
- The filtration coefficient for albumin is about 0.001, but about 7 g of albumin/day are filtered and taken up by the tubules and urine contains <30 mg albumin/day.

- Glomerular damage may cause excessive filtration of albumin and loss in the urine leading to hypoalbuminuria.
- Hypoalbuminuria leads to retention of sodium and water by activation of the renin–angiotensin–aldosterone system.
- The nephrotic syndrome is characterized by albuminuria, hypoalbuminaemia, gross oedema and hypercholesterolaemia.

ADDITIONAL READING

Braunwald E *et al.* (2001) *Harrison's Principles of Internal Medicine*, 15th edition. McGraw-Hill, New York.

Seldin DW & Giebisch G (2000) *The Kidney: Physiology and Pathophysiology*, 3rd edition. Lippincott Williams & Wilkins, Philadelphia.

Souhami RL & Moxham T (2002) *Textbook of Medicine*, 4th edition. Churchill Livingstone, London.

Whitworth JA & Lawrence JR (1994) *Textbook of Renal Disease*, 2nd edition. Churchill Livingstone, Edinburgh.

Shortness of breath in a smoker

CASE AND MCQS

Case introduction

Mr M.H. is a 50-year-old clerk who lost his job six months ago. Since that time he has been unemployed and at home. He is married with two adult children. He had childhood mumps and scarlet fever and had his tonsils removed at the age of 13. He has had no serious adult illnesses except for an attack of shingles 3 years ago.

He presents at the outpatient clinic complaining of breathlessness on exertion, together with a persistent pain-ful cough that produces white sputum. His breathlessness (dyspnoea) has been noticeable for just over 2 years and is not accompanied by pain in the legs or by deep chest pain suggestive of coronary insufficiency (angina pectoris). He claims to have smoked about two packs of cigarettes per day since he was 18 years old and to drink about three cans of beer daily.

Physical examination shows a somewhat overweight man (height 175 cm (5 ft 9 in), weight 86 kg (190 lb)) with laboured breathing and a deep-seated cough. His respiratory movements are pronounced and involve some accessory muscle activity. His chest is swollen in the anterior–posterior direction and auscultation reveals an expiratory wheeze. Examination of nails and face shows no evidence of cyanosis. Blood pressure is 140/85 mmHg, heart rate is 76 beats/min, oral temperature is 37.5°C.

Consider these features and make a preliminary diagnosis of the general type of disorder that is present.

 Q1 On the basis of the preliminary examination, Mr H.'s symptoms are most likely to be due to:

A. obstructive lung disease
B. restrictive lung disease
C. cardiac failure
D. essential hypertension
E. either A or C

Because his persistent productive cough suggests acute lower airways infection (bronchitis), you prescribe an antibiotic and arrange an appointment in a week's time for some respiratory function tests.

You start with the simplest quantitative tests of respiratory normality – measurement of static and kinetic lung volumes. The diagram in Fig. 8.1 is to remind you of how these parameters are defined. Abbreviations used are TLC – total lung capacity, FRC – functional residual capacity, IRV – inspiratory reserve volume, TV – tidal volume, FVC – forced vital capacity, FEV_1 – forced expiratory volume in one second, RV – residual volume.

Spirometry involves the patient breathing in and out while connected to a volume recorder. However, some of the components of lung volume illustrated above cannot be measured by spirometry.

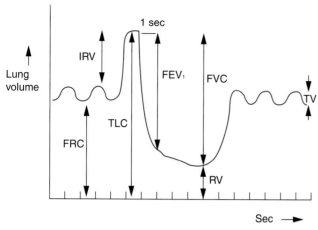

Fig. 8.1 Definitions of lung volumes as related to a spirometric recording.

Q2 The components that require additional forms of measurement include:

A. RV
B. FRC
C. TLC
D. all of the above
E. none of the above

Q3 Which of the following sets of measurements would be most informative in distinguishing between normal lung function, obstructive lung disease and restrictive lung disease?

A. FVC and TLC
B. FVC and IRV
C. FEV₁ and IRV
D. FEV₁ and FVC
E. FRC and TLC

The results of Mr H.'s lung volume testing are:

Total lung capacity (TLC)	6300 ml
Functional residual capacity (FRC)	4300 ml
Inspiratory reserve volume	1500 ml
Tidal volume (TV)	500 ml
Forced vital capacity (FVC)	3000 ml
Forced expiratory volume in one second (FEV₁)	1200 ml

Q4 Of these values, the following are within the normal range for an average-sized man:

A. all values
B. all values except FRC
C. all values except FVC
D. TLC, TV and IRV only
E. TLC and TV only

Q5 Using these data, an estimate of airways resistance would be most accurately obtained by comparison of:

A. TLC and FVC
B. FRC and FVC
C. FEV₁ and FVC
D. FEV₁ and TLC
E. FEV₁ and FRC

Q6 From this comparison, Mr H.'s absolute airways resistance is:

A. normal
B. about 50% of normal
C. about 150% of normal
D. about 200% of normal
E. cannot be calculated without more data

You use a peak flow meter to make some further measurements of his capacity to ventilate and obtain these data:

Resting minute ventilation	6.0 litres/min
Maximal minute ventilation	73 litres/min
Peak expiratory flow rate	170 litres/min
Peak inspiratory flow rate	220 litres/min

Q7 Which of these data are in the normal range?

A. resting minute ventilation
B. maximal minute ventilation
C. peak expiratory flow rate
D. peak inspiratory flow rate
E. none of them

Q8 Elevated airways resistance causes more dramatic reduction of peak expiratory than peak inspiratory flow rate because:

A. during inspiration, the negative intrathoracic pressure holds the airways open
B. during inspiration, the positive intrapleural pressure holds the airways open
C. during inspiration, the rise in intra-airways O_2 tension causes bronchodilation
D. during expiration, the rise in intra-airways CO_2 tension causes bronchoconstriction
E. none of the above

In summary, the respiratory function tests have shown that Mr H. has greatly elevated airways resistance (low FEV₁ and low peak ventilatory capacity), normal TLC but chronically inflated lungs (low IRV and high FRC). All these findings support the earlier physical evidence for an obstructive lung disease.

This conclusion is supported further by the flow/volume loop that you record with a pneumotachograph during a maximal inspiratory and expiratory effort. This shows an expiratory curve that is 'scooped-out' in shape by comparison with the normal pattern (Fig. 8.2).

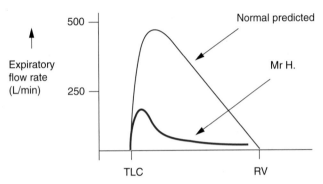

Fig. 8.2 A normal expiratory flow loop, and the corresponding recording obtained from M.H.

Q9 Increased small airways resistance results in a characteristic concave expiratory flow/volume curve because a rise in resistance to airflow:

A. causes rapid fatigue of expiratory muscles
B. reduces elastic recoil of the lung
C. increases elastic recoil of the lung
D. causes compression of the trachea
E. causes compression of the bronchioles

Now you need to decide whether Mr H. has active airways obstruction due to *asthma* or passive obstruction due to *emphysema* (often termed chronic obstructive pulmonary disease or COPD). Before we do this, let us review the main mechanisms that underlie these conditions.

Q10 The elevated airways resistance seen in patients with asthma is due to:

A. local oedema
B. stimulation of mucus secretion
C. bronchiolar smooth muscle contraction
D. all of the above
E. none of the above

Q11 In allergic (atopic) asthma, the trigger for elevated airways resistance is inhaled foreign proteins which:

A. stimulate mucosal chemoreceptors
B. cause degranulation of mast cells
C. increase interstitial oncotic pressure
D. create gap junctions between smooth muscle cells
E. induce a systemic inflammatory response

Q12 In non-atopic asthma, the trigger for elevated airways resistance is:

A. stimulation of mucosal chemoreceptors
B. degranulation of mast cells
C. increased interstitial oncotic pressure
D. gap junction formation between smooth muscle cells
E. a systemic inflammatory response

Q13 In emphysema, the elevated airways resistance is due mainly to:

A. increased alveolar wall surface tension
B. bronchiolar oedema
C. loss of intrapulmonary elastic tissue
D. accumulation of bronchiolar mucus
E. decreased elastic recoil of the lung

Approaches that may help in choosing between the alternatives of asthma and emphysema include chest X-ray, carbon monoxide transfer efficiency and blood gas analysis, but all these may give ambiguous results.

The simplest test is to check the efficacy of a bronchodilator drug. Since the airways obstruction in asthmatic patients is due primarily to active bronchoconstriction, a bronchodilator drug will restore ventilatory flow rates to nearly normal levels. In a patient with emphysema, whose airways obstruction is primarily structural, a bronchodilator agent has little effect.

You administer a beta-adrenoreceptor agonist (terbutaline) to Mr H. by aerosol and repeat the maximal ventilatory tests 5 minutes later. Peak expiratory flow rises from 170 to 220 litres/min, still only around 40% of the expected normal value. This confirms that the high airways resistance is not due to active bronchoconstriction but to passive compression of the airways typical of emphysema. What should your advice to the patient be?

First, although beta-adrenoreceptor stimulation had a relatively small effect on his ventilatory capacity, any bronchodilation must help reduce respiratory muscle work, so you prescribe him a terbutaline inhaler. Second, his condition is most probably caused (and certainly made worse) by his heavy smoking. You must advise him most strongly to stop smoking if he wishes his lung function not to deteriorate further.

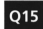 **Q14** **The trigger for chronic lung damage associated with smoking is:**

A. alveolar type II cell damage from smoke particles
B. obstruction of the alveolar surface by precipitated tars
C. pulmonary vasoconstriction by nicotine
D. constriction of the bronchioles by nicotine
E. paralysis of bronchial cilia by nicotine

Q15 **This effect of smoking leads to loss of intrapulmonary connective tissue because it results in:**

A. macrophagic invasion of the alveoli
B. bacterial destruction of alveolar type II cells
C. autoimmune attacks on alveolar type I cells
D. mismatching of ventilation and perfusion
E. none of the above

Six months later, Mr H. is brought to see you by his wife. He has been using his inhaler regularly but has continued to smoke as many cigarettes as previously. He is now clearly much sicker than when you last examined him:

- he appears confused
- his respiration is shallow, noisy and rapid (30 breaths/min)
- his blood pressure is 125/80 mmHg
- his pulse is 118 beats/min
- his oral temperature is 39.0°C
- his lips and nail beds appear slightly bluish (cyanotic).

Q16 **The appearance of cyanosis indicates that:**

A. arterial haemoglobin is at least 40% desaturated
B. arterial haemoglobin is at least 60% desaturated
C. at least 5 g/100 ml arterial haemoglobin is deoxygenated
D. at least 10 g/100 ml arterial haemoglobin is deoxygenated
E. at least 5 g/100 ml arterial haemoglobin is binding carbon dioxide

In view of his evident hypoxia, Mr H. is admitted. A transcutaneous pulse oximeter is clipped to his ear to continuously measure arterial haemoglobin saturation: at the time of admission the saturation is 70%. An arterial blood sample is taken for analysis and he is allowed to breathe spontaneously through a closely fitting facemask that supplies a constant concentration of 35% oxygen in air (Fig. 8.3a). In this type of mask, the central tube supplying oxygen is encased in another tube that is open to the air. Negative pressure created by the oxygen flow sucks air into the mask (the Venturi principle) at a rate that is determined by the aperture of the tube. This design allows more accurate regulation of oxygen content than is possible with a simple open mask (Fig. 8.3b). Even more

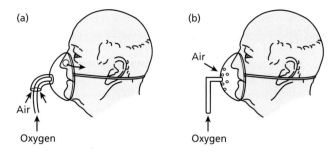

Fig. 8.3 Two types of mask used for oxygen supplementation of hypoxic patients.

importantly, the oxygen concentration that is delivered is independent of respiratory effort.

The following data come back from the lab from analysis of the blood sample taken at the time of admission:

Pa_{O_2}	55 mmHg (7.3 kPa)
Pa_{CO_2}	80 mmHg (11.0 kPa)
Arterial HCO_3^-	47 mmol/l

From these data, you can use the Henderson–Hasselbalch equation to calculate Mr H.'s arterial pH on admission. This equation states that $pH = 6.1 + \log_{10}[HCO_3^-]/[0.03.Pa_{CO_2}]$.

Q17 **Applying this equation, Mr H.'s arterial pH is:**

A. 7.25
B. 7.29
C. 7.35
D. 7.39
E. 7.50

Together with this information on arterial pH, you have absolute values for Pa_{CO_2} (83 mmHg or 11 kPa, normally 38–41 mmHg or 5.0–5.5 kPa) and arterial HCO_3^- (47 mmol/l, normally 22–30 mmol/l).

Q18 **Collectively, these data indicate that Mr H.'s acid–base status is:**

A. acute respiratory acidosis
B. acute metabolic acidosis
C. compensated respiratory acidosis
D. compensated metabolic acidosis
E. normal acid–base status

One hour after Mr H. has begun his oxygen therapy, you receive an urgent call from the ward reporting that his cyanosis is getting worse, not better, and that he is breathing less strongly. Haemoglobin saturation is now 50%.

What do you think has happened?

Q19 Respiratory depression as a result of breathing an elevated concentration of oxygen suggests that:

A. insufficient oxygen is being delivered to overcome the hypoxia
B. ventilatory drive is dependent on hypoxia receptors
C. the increased inspired oxygen is reducing central chemoreceptor drive
D. there is no chemoreceptor regulation of ventilation
E. there is CO_2 retention inside the mask

Q20 Under these circumstances, which of the following treatments would be most appropriate?

A. allow spontaneous ventilation
B. allow spontaneous ventilation and infuse isotonic $NaHCO_3$
C. ventilate with room air at twice minute volume
D. ventilate with room air at normal minute volume
E. ventilate with room air at normal minute volume and infuse isotonic $NaHCO_3$

Three hours after commencing the appropriate treatment, you find that Mr H. is alert, with a Pao_2 of 70 mmHg (9.3 kPa), $Paco_2$ of 45 mmHg (6.0 kPa) and an arterial pH of 7.41. Haemoglobin saturation is 85%.

He is discharged the next day, with strict instructions to stop smoking and with arrangements for weekly visits by a nurse to check his respiratory status. Following sputum culture, you give him a prescription for a suitable broad-spectrum antibiotic and also provide him with two other drugs that might help relieve his work of breathing.

Q21 From your knowledge of the autonomic control of airways function and the lung changes that characterize emphysema, which of the following pharmacological approaches might be useful adjuncts to beta-adrenoreceptor agonists in reducing Mr H.'s airways resistance?

A. glucocorticoids, muscarinic receptor antagonists and alpha-adrenoreceptor antagonists
B. glucocorticoids, muscarinic receptor antagonists and phosphodiesterase inhibitors
C. glucocorticoids, muscarinic receptor agonists and phosphodiesterase inhibitors
D. glucocorticoids, muscarinic receptor agonists and alpha-adrenoreceptor antagonists
E. glucocorticoids, muscarinic receptor antagonists and mast cell stabilizers

As well as pharmacological treatment, there are other approaches that can be used to reduce the discomfort in the patient with severe emphysema.

Q22 Think about patients in Mr H.'s situation and see if you can identify two ways in which surgical interventions might be beneficial.

MCQ ANSWERS AND FEEDBACK

1.A. A distended thoracic cage at rest, an expiratory wheeze and a history of intrapulmonary cough all suggest partial airway obstruction. Chest distension would not be expected with restrictive disease since by definition thoracic expansion would be less than usual, and an expiratory wheeze is uncommon in restrictive disease. Cardiac failure could cause effort-dependent limitation to gas exchange because of pulmonary oedema. However, since both blood pressure and resting heart rate suggest normal cardiac function, this is not the most likely option.

2.D. Spirometry can only measure *volume changes* within the lung during the respiratory cycle. Since even after maximal expiration there is still a substantial volume of air left in the lung (the RV), none of the components of lung volume that include this residual air can be quantified using spirometry.

The easiest way to quantify RV, FRC and TLC is to have the patient breathe a known concentration of an inert gas such as helium and to measure the dilution of this gas in the lung.

3.D. The proportion of FVC that can be blown out over the first second of a maximal expiratory effort (that is, the FEV_1) is reduced below normal when the airways are partially obstructed. In restrictive lung disease due to muscle weakness or ribcage deformation, $FEV_1 : FVC$ is normal; in restrictive disease due to intrapulmonary rigidity (caused for example by scar tissue), the ratio is actually increased because of increased elastic recoil. In both obstructive and restrictive states, the absolute volumes of both FEV_1 and FVC will be considerably less than that predicted from the patient's body size. Although the absolute magnitudes of the other parameters mentioned may be abnormal in patients with lung disease, they cannot provide information that would simultaneously distinguish normality and the two different disease types.

4.E. In a normal individual, you would expect resting ventilatory movements to be set at around the midpoint of lung expansion, so IRV should be about the same volume as FRC. A maximal expiratory movement normally compresses the lung down to a volume of around 1–1.3 litres, representing the minimum size to which the ribcage can collapse, so FVC should be around 5000 ml (6300 minus 1300). Since almost all of this air can normally be blown out during the first second of forced expiration, FEV_1 should be much greater than 1400 ml.

5.C. As FEV_1 is the only parameter that reflects the rate of air movement, it is essential for interpreting resistance to flow. However, in order to derive a value that can be used to assess normality independent of lung size, the volume of air moved per unit time must be related to the total volume available for expiration. The standard index used is therefore FEV_1:FVC%.

6.D. In normal individuals, FEV_1 is reproducibly 80–85% of FVC, so Mr H.'s FEV_1:FVC of [1200:3000] or 40% shows that resistance to flow is about twice normal.

7.A. Even substantial elevation of airways resistance may not reduce minute ventilation at rest, although in order to overcome the resistance Mr H. must do much more respiratory muscle work than normal. The limiting effect of elevated resistance to flow becomes obvious when he attempts to ventilate maximally; then we see a peak inspiratory flow rate that is about 60% of the normal value and peak expiratory flow rate that is only around 30% normal.

8.A. The bronchiolar responses to intraluminal gas tensions, with bronchodilation in response to elevated P_{CO_2} or reduced P_{O_2}, are important in optimizing regional ventilation/perfusion matching. However, they do not occur rapidly enough to cause fluctuations in airways resistance during one respiratory cycle.

9.E. When the lung is distended, the elastic connective tissue elements are stretched taut. This helps to hold the smaller airways open against the external compression caused by expiratory muscle contraction. As expiration continues and lung volume falls, the connective tissue becomes less taut and so the airways are more compressed. This causes a progressive decline in flow rate. The decline is much more pronounced when there is pre-existing elevation of airways resistance, because absolute flow resistance depends on absolute tube diameter (remember Poiseuille's law?). Since the effect of increased resistance is much more pronounced at submaximal lung vol-

umes, measuring maximum flow rates at 25% and 50% TLC is a more sensitive indicator of obstructive disease than measurements of FEV_1 or peak expiratory flow rate alone.

10.D. Regardless of the triggering stimuli, the bronchiolar wall in a patient with acute asthma typically shows local vasodilation and extravasation of fluid, increased mucus secretion and contraction of the smooth musculature.

11.B. Atopic asthma is triggered by an IgE-mediated response to foreign protein, most commonly pollen or particles of animal skin or saliva. IgE molecules dock on mast cells and the antigen–antibody reaction causes release from the mast cell of several chemical factors (including histamine, leukotrienes and prostaglandins) into the local environment. These collectively relax arteriolar smooth muscle, increase capillary permeability, activate mucus gland secretion and cause bronchiolar smooth muscle contraction.

12.A. The stimulus for non-atopic asthma is usually inhalation of a chemical vapour that activates irritant receptors in the airway mucosa, Specific chemical moieties include sulphur and nitrogen dioxides from motor exhaust, sulphur dioxide in soft drinks and preserved foods and ozone generated by photochemical reactions. Irritant receptor activation causes reflex stimulation of vagal motor neurons that supply the bronchiolar mucous glands and smooth musculature.

This vagal reflex seems to be abnormally sensitive in many patients with atopic asthma as well as in the non-atopic group. For example, inhaling cold dry air tends to dry out the airway mucosa and activate the irritant receptors. This response is seen in many asthmatics as an acute attack of asthma during exercise, which can be prevented if the individual breathes warm, humid air.

13.C. The primary change in lung structure that characterizes emphysema is the loss of intrapulmonary connective tissue, resulting in airways that are far more easily compressed by expiratory pressures than those in a normal lung. Nevertheless, additional reduction of airways diameter by local inflammatory responses to infection (bronchitis) is undoubtedly an accompanying feature in most patients with smoking-related emphysema. The reduced elastic recoil caused by loss of connective tissue contributes to increased FRC and reduced IRC and substantially increases the amount of muscle work needed for expiratory movements, but does not by itself affect resistance to flow.

14.E. The layer of secreted mucus lining the airways traps most inhaled particulate matter and continual ciliary activity is essential for this contaminated mucus to be cleared from the airways into the nose and mouth. When the cilia are paralysed, much of the mucus instead falls into the alveoli, where it constitutes an ideal culture medium for bacterial infection. Inhalation of high concentrations of some types of toxic smoke, as may occur during firefighting, can directly damage type II cells and cause physical obstruction of the alveolar exchange surface. However, the toxicity of cigarette smoke is insufficient to produce direct damage. Nicotine absorbed directly into the airway wall stimulates intramural vagal ganglia and causes measurable bronchoconstriction during an episode of smoking, but this effect wears off within 15–20 minutes after the cigarette is finished.

15.A. Macrophages are continually traversing all organs in search of foreign or damaged cells that should be phagocytosed. So recurrent alveolar infection will be associated with macrophages moving through the pulmonary parenchyma over a long period. In order to penetrate through a tissue, macrophages need to create local pathways for themselves. They achieve this by secreting proteases that digest intercellular connective tissue. In solid organs, these holes are rapidly repaired and do not alter the internal organ structure. In lung, on the other hand, because the connective tissue strands are stretched though space, they retract when one end is detached and cannot be repaired effectively.

16.C. The presence of 5 g of deoxygenated haemoglobin per 100 ml blood is sufficient to make the blood appear blue rather than red. In arterial blood and in the capillary blood that is visible through the skin, cyanosis usually signifies substantially reduced oxygen transport. But this is not always the case. Arterial blood would also appear cyanotic if there was a normal amount of oxygenated haemoglobin plus an additional 5 g/100 ml of deoxygenated haemoglobin.

17.D. A ratio of 20:1 (= antilog$_{10}$1.3) between plasma bicarbonate (mmol/l) and P_{CO_2} (mmHg × 0.03) will under stable conditions provide a pH of 7.4 regardless of the actual levels of these substances. If you need to calculate pH using data on proton concentration rather than components of the carbonic acid system, then you can use the equation pH = $-\log_{10}[H^+]$. Thus, pH 7.00 would be represented by a proton concentration of 100 nmol/l.

18.C. In acute respiratory acidosis there is retention of excess plasma CO_2 but there has not yet been time for renal compensation to occur. If both P_{aCO_2} and bicarbonate are elevated, this indicates that compensatory adjustments have had time to take place. In different reference texts you will find slightly different absolute minimal and maximal values quoted for normal plasma bicarbonate, with limits ranging between 20 mmol/l and 32 mmol/l. This variability is partly because some sources ignore the rare outlying values and partly because many blood analysis machines calculate two values for bicarbonate: one based on pH and measured CO_2 levels and one based on pH and a standard 'normal' level of CO_2. However, you can be confident that anything outside the range 20–32 mmol/l is definitely not compatible with normal acid–base status.

19.B. Extreme hypercapnia is a constant concern in patients whose respiratory exchange function has been depressed over a prolonged period. Continual retention of carbon dioxide often leads eventually to desensitization of the central chemoreceptors, so further rises in P_{aCO_2} are not detected and therefore do not stimulate respiratory drive. In these patients, peripheral chemoreceptor activation due to arterial hypoxia is the primary chemical stimulus to ventilation, leading to the paradox that gas exchange becomes less efficient when the patient is less deprived of oxygen. In Mr H.'s case, analysis of an arterial sample taken just before his oxygen supplementation was terminated showed a P_{aO_2} of 45 mmHg (6.0 kPa) and a P_{aCO_2} of 90 mmHg (12 kPa).

Occasionally, retention of CO_2 can occur in hospital when the patient is fitted with a tight-fitting facemask designed to deliver near-atmospheric concentrations of oxygen, but this could not occur with the mask used in Mr H.'s case.

20.D. It is clear from the blood gas values on admission that Mr H.'s hypoxia is not sufficient to endanger oxygenation of his tissues – with a P_{aO_2} of 55 mmHg (7.3 kPa) his haemoglobin is still 70% saturated. Therefore, the most immediate concern has to be reversal of his pronounced hypercapnia. Normal lung expansion with room air will automatically create an effective gradient for diffusion into the alveolar air. Increasing the tidal volume above normal would improve this gradient but, in a patient with reduced intrapulmonary connective tissue, it might also cause traumatic damage to the lung. The absence of adequate spontaneous ventilatory movements is due to progressive retention of CO_2 to the extent that it is inhibiting central respiratory drive; this problem will not be remedied by adding more bicarbonate to the bloodstream.

21.B. Inhibiting the action of vagal bronchoconstrictor nerves with a muscarinic receptor antagonist improves airways conductance in some patients with emphysema. These individuals, like some asthmatics, may have hypersensitive mucosal irritant receptors and so be at risk of reflex vagal bronchoconstriction. Methylxanthines such as aminophylline can be effective bronchodilators because they inhibit phosphodiesterase and therefore increase cyclic AMP levels in the bronchiolar smooth muscle cells. About 20% of patients also improve when given anti-inflammatory corticosteroids such as prednisolone, probably because in these cases bronchitis is contributing to overall airways resistance.

22. When lung function is very severely compromised, lung transplantation is occasionally an option, but donor organs are very scarce. Another surgical strategy that could be considered is the counter-intuitive approach of surgically removing some lung tissue. The logic is that removal of non-functional lung will not reduce gas exchange, but will allow the remaining tissue to expand further, increasing its elastic recoil and helping to hold the airways open during expiration. In practice, the operation is only suited to a minority of patients and has a relatively high mortality rate, but it is an interesting example of how knowledge of pathophysiology leads to innovations in patient care.

CASE REVIEW

Mr H. had been coughing and experiencing exertional dyspnoea for years before he first came to see you. You may wonder why he waited until his disease was so advanced before seeking help. In fact, because emphysemic loss of lung tissue occurs so slowly and because of the large normal respiratory reserve, people with a sedentary lifestyle often do not notice any disturbance of respiratory function until a large proportion of their lung has been destroyed. Many smokers are also reluctant to seek help as soon as they should, because they know that they will be advised to give up smoking.

Apart from that advice, which is of limited use because of nicotine addiction, what strategies are available to help a patient with emphysema? The primary aim must be to keep airways resistance as low as possible and the beta-adrenoreceptor agonist drugs are the mainstay of this strategy. The sensation of breathlessness, which is one of the most distressing aspects of emphysema from the patients' point of view, is caused by respiratory muscle fatigue and any reduction in absolute airways resistance will reduce respiratory muscle work. So bronchodilation provides a substantial benefit for a patient's quality of life, even though it improves gas exchange only very little.

As indicated in Question 21, a variety of additional pharmacological approaches are often used. These include inhibiting the effects of vagal bronchoconstrictor nerves with antimuscarinic agents, enhancing bronchiolar dilation by inhibiting intracellular phosphodiesterase and decreasing mucosal inflammatory reactions with corticosteroids. However, the effects of all these agents are variable and they provide long-term benefits over what would be achieved with a beta-adrenoreceptor agonist alone only in relatively small subgroups of patients.

In patients whose emphysema is so severe that they have limited mobility, low-dose oxygen administration via nasal prongs on a virtually continuous basis will help them to remain ambulatory. Some of these patients will also benefit from a gentle aerobic training programme, which probably improves their exercise tolerance by increasing skeletal muscle capillarization.

Unfortunately, there is nothing you can do to *reverse* the disease process of emphysema. If Mr H. stops smoking this will slow his lung deterioration, but nothing can repair the structural damage or stop the further loss of respiratory function that will occur inevitably with age. Broad-spectrum antibiotic treatment at the first sign of a respiratory infection will help prevent (or at least delay) the worst scenario of hypercapnic respiratory failure and pneumonia, although continual antibiotic cover would be counterproductive because of bacterial resistance. Nevertheless, the realistic assessment must be that a patient such as Mr H. will inevitably have progressive reduction in mobility with a likely terminal stage of being bed-ridden and reliant on supplementary O_2.

KEY POINTS

- The chronic lung disease associated with smoking is due primarily to loss of the intrapulmonary connective tissue that holds the airways open during expiration and provides the property of elastic recoil.
- This damage is irreversible, so emphysema cannot be cured.
- As well, bronchodilator drugs have much less therapeutic effect than in obstructive disease caused by asthma.

- Sustained retention of excess carbon dioxide often desensitizes the central chemoreceptors.
- In these hypercapnic patients, much of the respiratory drive is from peripheral hypoxia receptors.
- The reliance of spontaneous ventilation on absolute plasma oxygen levels must be considered when reversing hypoxia.

ADDITIONAL READING

Benditt JO (2004) Surgical therapies for chronic obstructive pulmonary disease. *Respiratory Care* **49**: 53–63.

Burge S (2001) Should inhaled corticosteroids be used in the long term treatment of chronic obstructive pulmonary disease? *Drugs* **61**: 1535–44.

Clancy LJ (1977) Assessment of the hypoxic drive to breathing in normal man and the effects and treatment of hypoxia in patients with chronic bronchitis and emphysema. *Irish Journal of Medical Science* **146**: 226–31.

Petty TL (2002) COPD in perspective. *Chest* **121**: 116S–120S.

The Global Initiative for Chronic Obstructive Lung Disease website (currently http://www.goldcopd.com/).

Chest pain on exercise

CASE AND MCQS

Case introduction

Mr S.O'R. presents at your surgery complaining of increasing breathlessness, with chest pain on exertion and episodes of fainting. He is a 64-year-old man who is self-employed as a motor dealer. He says he smokes about 20 cigarettes per day and drinks moderately. His father died of a heart attack at the age of 65 and his mother is still alive, aged 91. He has no memories of serious illnesses except for childhood mumps and measles.

Twelve months ago he began to notice breathlessness when playing tennis. Since that time he has become progressively more breathless during exercise and sometimes feels dizzy. Over the past few weeks, he is out of breath when walking more than about 20 m (65 ft) without rest and has pain in his chest if he tries to hurry.

Several times over the last month he has felt faint when standing up suddenly. He has now come to see you because, last night, he fainted when he got out of bed to urinate.

Q1 On the basis of this preliminary information, the primary cause of Mr O'R.'s low exercise tolerance seems most likely to be:

A. limited coronary perfusion
B. limited cardiac output
C. limited gas exchange
D. defective baroreflex function
E. a mixture of respiratory and circulatory problems

When Mr O'R. has rested supine on your couch for 10 minutes, his brachial blood pressure is 116/88 mmHg and his pulse rate is 70 beats/min. Consider whether or not these values are what you would expect for a normal cardiovascular system.

Q2 Given the patient's resting heart rate, are any of the blood pressure parameters outside the normal range?

A. systolic pressure
B. diastolic pressure
C. mean arterial pressure
D. pulse pressure
E. all blood pressure values are within the normal range

You now go on to record Mr O'R.'s ECG and take a blood sample for analysis. The resulting ECG record is shown in Fig. 9.1.

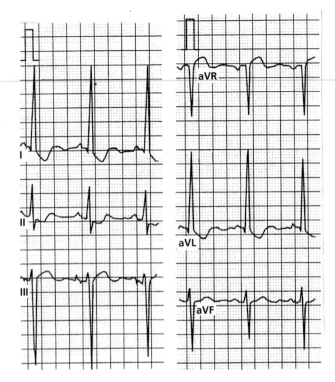

Fig. 9.1 Portion of a 12-lead ECG recorded from Mr O'R. on initial examination, showing waveforms for leads I–III and aVR, aVL and aVF.

Analysis of the blood sample you took shows the following values:

Sodium	140 mmol/l
Calcium	2.1 mmol/l
Bicarbonate	26 mmol/l
Potassium	4.8 mmol/l
Chloride	98 mmol/l
Cholesterol	6.4 mmol/l

Q5 These data indicate:

A. hypocalcaemia
B. hyperkalaemia
C. metabolic alkalosis
D. hypercholesterolaemia
E. normal values for all data

You take Mr O'R.'s pulse and listen to his chest. The radial and carotid pulses are relatively weak and seem to be less sharp (that is, less abrupt in onset) than you would expect in a normal person. There is a pronounced murmur associated with the first heart sound. This murmur lasts almost until the second heart sound and is poorly localized. The second sound seems normal.

Q6 The timing and characteristics of the first heart sound provide useful information on the efficiency of cardiac function, because the event that produces the dominant part of the sound is:

A. opening of the atrioventricular valves
B. fast ventricular filling
C. closing of the atrioventricular valves
D. fast ventricular ejection
E. closing of the semi-lunar valves

Q3 This ECG indicates:

A. normal sequence of cardiac excitation
B. complete heart block
C. left bundle branch block
D. incomplete heart block
E. atrial fibrillation

Q4 From the waveform amplitudes and comparison of the records taken from different leads, you can conclude that the heart is:

A. vertical and normal
B. vertical with right ventricular hypertrophy
C. vertical with left ventricular hypertrophy
D. horizontal with right ventricular hypertrophy
E. horizontal with left ventricular hypertrophy

Q7 At this stage of investigation, you can conclude that the patient's symptoms of breathlessness, angina and syncope are definitely not due to:

A. pulmonary valve stenosis
B. mitral valve regurgitation
C. aortic valve stenosis
D. tricuspid valve regurgitation
E. aortic valve regurgitation

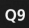 **Q8** Using only non-invasive examination of a patient, how could you distinguish between mitral regurgitation and tricuspid regurgitation?

With this background of non-invasive information, it would be helpful to obtain some quantitative measurements of cardiac function in order to determine the basis of Mr O.R.'s reduced cardiac reserve.

You arrange for him to attend the catheter lab in the local cardiology department. A Swan–Ganz catheter is inserted via the right jugular vein through his right heart and into a main pulmonary artery. Pressures are recorded at these different sites and the catheter is then passed downstream into a small pulmonary artery so as to be able to record pulmonary wedge pressure.

The data obtained are as follows:

Right atrial pressure	4/0 mmHg
Right ventricular pressure	24/0 mmHg
Pulmonary arterial pressure	23/14 mmHg
Pulmonary wedge pressure	14/11 mmHg

 Q9 Pulmonary wedge pressure provides a measurement of:

A. left ventricular pressure
B. left atrial pressure
C. pulmonary capillary pressure
D. pulmonary arterial pressure
E. pulmonary gas exchange

Q10 The pressure recordings indicate that at least one of the possible causes that were identified in Question 7 can be excluded. Which can be excluded?

A. pulmonary stenosis
B. mitral regurgitation
C. tricuspid regurgitation
D. aortic stenosis
E. both A and C

In order to resolve the exact site of damage, a catheter is passed retrogradely under radiographic guidance from the femoral artery into the left ventricle and is then withdrawn into the aorta, while pressure is recorded continuously. The resulting pressure recordings (Fig. 9.2) show a left intraventricular pressure of 190/10 mmHg and an aortic pressure of 120/86 mmHg.

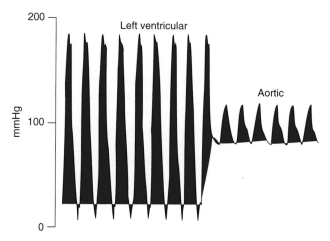

Fig. 9.2 Pressure recordings from Mr O'R.'s left ventricle and aorta.

Q11 Do these data indicate that the problem is due to an incompetent mitral valve or to a stenosed aortic valve?

The diagnosis is confirmed by echocardiography. You will remember that the original symptoms that Mr O'R. complained of were:
- breathlessness on exertion
- angina on exertion
- syncope on standing.

Let us consider these again, in the context of the established diagnosis.

Q12 Mr O'R.'s exertional breathlessness is caused by:

A. hypercapnia due to poor muscle perfusion
B. hypercapnia due to elevated pulmonary venous pressure
C. metabolic acidosis due to poor muscle perfusion
D. reduced space for lung expansion due to cardiac hypertrophy
E. none of the above

Q13 Mr O'R.'s exertional angina is caused by:

A. decreased pulmonary oxygen uptake due to increased pulmonary venous pressure
B. decreased washout of myocardial metabolites due to reduced peak coronary perfusion
C. decreased washout of myocardial metabolites due to reduced time for coronary perfusion
D. both B and C
E. all of A, B and C

Q14 Mr O'R.'s faintness on standing is caused by:

A. inability to produce baroreflex vasoconstriction because there is already maximal sympathetic drive
B. inability to increase cardiac output because of the high output resistance
C. absence of baroreceptor activation because of low arterial pulse pressure
D. reduced venous return because of high pulmonary venous pressure
E. both B and C

Q15 Mr O'R.'s symptoms will be helped by:

A. a beta-adrenoreceptor antagonist to slow his heart rate and improve ventricular filling
B. an alpha-adrenoreceptor agonist to cause peripheral vasoconstriction
C. an abdominal corset to mobilize pooled splanchnic blood
D. an alpha-adrenoreceptor antagonist to cause peripheral vasodilation
E. none of the above

Insertion of a prosthetic valve is the only effective long-term treatment for this condition. However, it will not be possible to find Mr O'R. a surgical bed for some months. In the meantime, care must be taken to prevent any exacerbation of his problem. One major concern is that his left ventricular endocardium is being continually subjected to excessive turbulence. This tends to damage the endocardial cells and sensitize them to infective organisms. Antibiotic cover must therefore be given in this type of patient if there is a risk of access of bacteria to the circulation (for example during invasive dental procedures).

Two months later, you see Mr O'R. again. His condition has deteriorated noticeably over this period.

- He is now breathless even with very mild exertion.
- He becomes dyspnoeic if he lies down during the night (*nocturnal orthopnoea*), so that he has to sleep with several pillows.
- He also becomes dizzy when standing, much more often then he did before.
- His blood pressure at rest is now 110/88 mmHg.
- His pulse rate is 42 beats/min.
- Chest auscultation shows that his systolic murmur now persists throughout systole.
- The murmur is continuous with the second heart sound.
- It is not as loud as when you assessed it originally.
- On chest palpation, you can detect a vibration during systole (a *thrill*).
- The thrill can also be felt over the common carotid artery, especially on the right side.
  An ECG recording shows the pattern in Fig. 9.3.

Q16 This ECG shows that Mr O'R.'s bradycardia at rest is due to:

A. first degree atrioventricular block
B. second degree atrioventricular block
C. complete atrioventricular block
D. bundle branch block
E. sinus bradycardia

Q17 From the absolute heart rate and appearance of the QRS complex, the location of the pacemaker driving ventricular excitation is:

A. the atrioventricular node
B. the atrioventricular pathway
C. bundle of His
D. bundle branch
E. ventricular muscle

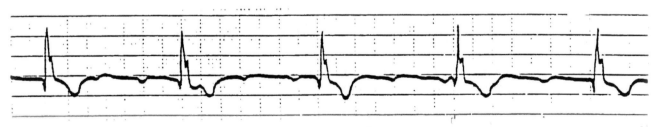

Fig. 9.3 Mr O'R.'s ECG (lead II) on his return visit.

The increased symptoms, together with the fact that his ejection murmur now persists throughout systole, indicate that Mr O'R.'s stenosis is rapidly becoming more severe. This will impose a progressively greater left ventricular workload which is increased further by the large end-diastolic ventricular volume and pressure caused by his low heart rate.

A substantially increased cardiac workload at rest always carries the dangers of a patient developing cardiac failure and pulmonary oedema.

> **Q18** From your knowledge of forces that regulate transcapillary water movement, what will be the lowest left atrial pressure that is likely to initiate pulmonary oedema?

A. 15 mmHg
B. 20 mmHg
C. 25 mmHg
D. 35 mmHg
E. 60 mmHg

Mr O'R. is prescribed a diuretic until the time of operation. This will lower his blood volume and so reduce cardiac work. The agent chosen is one of the thiazide class of diuretics, which provide a smaller degree of water loss than is produced by some other types of diuretic agent.

> **Q19** Thiazide diuretics:

A. act by inhibition of carbonic anhydrase
B. act on the distal tubule
C. decrease potassium excretion
D. act on the loop of Henle
E. antagonize the action of aldosterone

Five weeks later, Mr O'R. is given an aortic valve prosthesis. The type is a ball-and-cage design known as the Starr–Edwards valve. An X-ray image of the implanted valve is shown in Fig. 9.4. Note the circular rim of the valve seated in the aortic orifice and the loop of the cage above it. Because the ball valve inside the cage is plastic, it does not show up as opaque on the X-ray.

At operation, two cusps of his aortic valve are found to be infiltrated with calcium deposits, so that they have been able

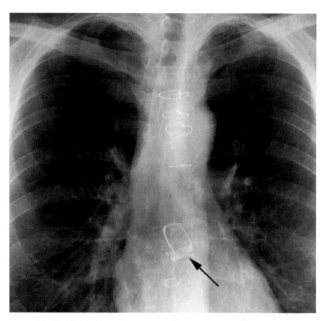

Fig. 9.4 Frontal X-ray of Mr O'R.'s chest after insertion of his aortic valve prosthesis. The implant is arrowed.

to open only slightly during systole. It is likely that the atrioventricular block that developed prior to the operation was caused by a second calcium deposit pressing on the conducting tissue of the atrioventricular node. It would not be technically feasible, however, to try to remove that deposit, so pacing is the only way in which full cardiac function can be restored. A pacemaker is implanted of a type that delivers separately timed impulses for activation of atria and ventricles, thus allowing resynchronization of atrial and ventricular pumping.

The presence of an artifical valve leads frequently to generation of intravascular clots (*thrombi*). It is therefore important for Mr O'R. to be given continual anticoagulant cover post-operatively. The drug chosen is warfarin.

> **Q20** The anticoagulant action of warfarin:

A. is often reduced in patients taking antibiotics
B. involves inhibition of binding of vitamin K to an apoenzyme
C. affects only the intrinsic clotting pathway
D. involves inactivation of thrombin
E. mimics the clotting defect seen in haemophilia

MCQ ANSWERS AND FEEDBACK

1.B. Mechanical limitation of ventricular ability to pump blood would limit the patient's capacity to raise cardiac output during exercise and postural change. This would in turn limit gas exchange, blood pressure control and coronary perfusion. Deficient coronary perfusion would explain the chest pain (*angina*) but would not explain the breathlessness (*dyspnoea*), while lung disease would explain the dyspnoea but not the angina. Defective baroreflex function might cause fainting, but cannot account for the breathlessness, which suggests some mismatch between respiratory drive and its effectiveness in maintaining normal blood gases. There could be a mixture of respiratory and circulatory problems, but it is simplest for a start to assume that both respiratory and circulatory symptoms are caused by the same underlying problem.

2.D. Pulse pressure is very low considering that heart rate is at a normal resting value and that therefore there is plenty of time for ventricular filling. In a normal individual at rest, you would expect a pulse pressure of at least 40 mmHg with a heart rate around 70 beats/min. Although systolic and mean blood pressures are rather low for an individual of Mr O'R.'s age, and diastolic pressure is relatively high, none of these values are outside the range of values that you might find in a normal population.

3.A. This ECG may not look entirely normal but it shows a normal sequence of excitation. Each QRS complex is preceded by a P wave, so there cannot be atrial fibrillation or a defect in atrioventricular node conduction. The QRS complex is also less than 100 ms in duration and of normal shape, so there must be normal conduction of impulses through the intraventricular conducting system; therefore bundle branch block can be excluded.

4.E. With a normal amount of ventricular muscle tissue, the R wave is never greater than 2.5 mV in any lead. The R waves in this recording are up to 3 mV or more, indicating a substantial degree of ventricular hypertrophy. This is at least predominantly on the left side because chest leads V_1–V_2 show large negative R waves. If the hypertrophy were on the right side, you would expect only small negative or even positive R waves in these leads. It is worth noting, however, that hypertrophy of both ventricles is often difficult to distinguish from simple left-sided hypertrophy.

Frontal plane rotation of the heart can be deduced from the pattern of QRS variation between the different frontal leads. With a vertical heart (= right axis deviation) the mean QRS vector is oriented to the left and inferiorly (+75 to +110 degrees), which results in the R waves being positive in aVF and negative in aVL and aVR. A horizontal heart (= left axis deviation) has a mean vector orientation to the left and superiorly (0–130 degrees), so the R waves are negative in aVR and aVF and positive in aVL. Although normal individuals show a wide range of frontal orientations, left ventricular hypertrophy typically shifts the heart towards a more horizontal position – that is, produces more left axis deviation.

5.D. None of the electrolytes are outside the normal range of variability, but a plasma cholesterol level of 5.0 mmol/l

(200 mg/dl) or less is recommended for cardiovascular health. In terms of clinical interpretation, the cholesterol concentration by itself is of limited value. It is more important to know in what form most of this cholesterol is carried in the plasma. Cholesterol bound to high-density lipoprotein (HDL) represents cholesterol that is being recycled from tissue cells to hepatic metabolism, while the proportion bound to low-density lipoprotein (LDL) is cholesterol that is being transported to tissue cells. Since deposition of cholesterol in arterial walls seems to be the initiating stage of atherosclerosis, current thinking is that the ratio of plasma LDL:HDL is a better indicator of cardiovascular risk than the total amount of circulating cholesterol (see also Case 13).

6.C. In a normal heart, the first sound lasts from the beginning of isovolumetric ventricular contraction to about the moment of semi-lunar valve opening (that is, the beginning of ventricular ejection). The sound results from vibrations in the walls and contents of the ventricles, set up by atrioventricular valve closure and rebound of the stretched chordae tendineae. This sequence of events causes the initial loud part of the first sound. A softer component of the sound may continue during the first 20–40 ms of ejection, due to intraventricular turbulence caused by the rapid acceleration of blood through the aortic orifice.

7.E. If the aortic valve does not shut fully at the end of systole, some of the pressurized blood in the aorta will flow back into the left ventricle during diastole rather than flowing downstream through the arteries. If the amount of backflow is sufficient, this will cause a diastolic murmur but, more importantly, it cannot be associated with a systolic murmur. A further point that excludes aortic regurgitation is that the backflow of blood from aorta to ventricle would cause diastolic blood pressure to be lower than normal, so that the pulse pressure would be increased: Mr O'R.'s pulse pressure is abnormally narrow. Each of the remaining alternatives would be associated with a systolic murmur and reduced ventricular ejection, so none can be absolutely excluded at this time.

8. Incompetence of either set of atrioventricular valves will cause regurgitation of ventricular blood during systole, with an associated systolic murmur, reduced stroke volume and reduced pulse pressure. However, tricuspid regurgitation into the right atrium will also cause a rise in central venous pressure during systole, which can be detected by observation of the jugular pulse wave. In theory, left and right regurgitation can also be distinguished by auscultation, as the areas of the chest wall at which murmurs are heard most clearly are slightly different for mitral and tricuspid valves. But because both valves are deep in the heart and the sounds are diffused through the ventricular walls before reaching the surface of the chest, this distinction is not always possible in practice.

9.B. Pulmonary wedge pressure is measured by passing an open-tipped catheter from the right side of the heart into the pulmonary arterial tree until it jams in a small artery. Under these circumstances, the catheter can record pressures from downstream only and, because of the very low longitudinal resistance of the pulmonary vascular bed, the pressure recorded approximates the pressure in the left atrium. This technique is the only practicable way of obtaining a quantitative index of left atrial pressure, because it is not technically possible to pass a catheter retrogradely into the atrium from the left ventricle.

10.E. Stenosis of the pulmonary valve would impose a resistance on ejection of blood from the right heart, so systolic pressure would be lower in pulmonary artery than in right ventricle. If the tricuspid valve were incompetent, it would not close fully during systole. This would elevate systolic right atrial pressure towards the value generated in the right ventricle. The peak value of 4 mmHg shown is normal for right atrium, so the tricuspid valve must be patent. The pumping defect must therefore be located in the left heart and this is supported by the high left atrial pressure (normally around 6/2 mmHg). Such a situation could be explained by defective closure of the mitral valve with backflow of blood during systole, or by defective opening of the aortic valve leading to accumulation of blood in both left atrium and left ventricle.

11. The marked pressure gradient between ventricle and aorta indicates a high resistance to flow across this junction, consistent with the aortic valve not opening fully. Failure of the mitral valve to shut during ventricular contraction would reduce stroke volume because some blood would be ejected backwards into the left atrium, but it could not produce a difference between ventricular and aortic pressures.

12.C. The subjective symptom of breathlessness is related to respiratory muscle fatigue. This is caused usually by excessive chemoreceptor drive related to acid–base imbalance or to hypoxia. The most likely scenario in Mr O'R.'s case is that poor delivery of oxygenated blood during exercise leads to increased muscle reliance on anaerobic metabolism. This results in elevation of plasma lactate, with consequent stimulation of the proton-sensitive peripheral chemoreceptors. An additional contribution to respiratory muscle fatigue would be the inability of the left heart to empty adequately because of the high outflow resistance. This will increase pulmonary venous pressure, distending the lung and lowering its elasticity. Ventilating a less elastic lung requires more respiratory muscle work.

13.D. Angina is a good indicator of insufficient coronary blood flow. It is due to activation of chemosensitive pain fibres by interstitial accumulation of myocardial metabolites that are normally washed away in the bloodstream. This patient's capacity to increase coronary blood flow during exercise is limited both by his low stroke volume and by the fact that left coronary perfusion is reduced by the prolonged high myocardial pressure generated during systole.

14.B. The fall in venous return caused by gravitational venous pooling on standing normally initiates a reflex rise in peripheral resistance via vasoconstriction and a reflex increase in cardiac output via tachycardia. In the presence of a stenosed aortic valve, the second part of this response is ineffective, so it is more difficult to maintain blood pressure accurately over the first few seconds of standing. Mechanoreceptive nerve endings such as those in the baroreceptor regions do react to phasic shifts in stimulus as well as to a steady state stimulus, but the average pressure across the entire pulse wave is more important than pulse pressure magnitude in initiating baroreflex responses.

15.E. In this patient, bradycardia will not substantially increase stroke volume, because of the limitations imposed by the high outflow resistance. In fact, since bradycardia will increase the duration of systole, it may have the adverse effect of increasing coronary insufficiency and angina. Changes in peripheral resistance caused by drug administration will also be ineffective. Generalized vasoconstriction will elevate peripheral resistance and make it more difficult for the left ventricle to eject an adequate stroke volume, while generalized vasodilation will make it more difficult to maintain an adequate perfusion pressure gradient for peripheral vascular perfusion. Mobilizing pooled splanchnic blood will not increase cardiac output so long as ventricular outflow resistance remains so high, because the mobilized blood will just redistribute to some other compliant area such as the pulmonary veins.

16.C. As regular P waves can be seen at a frequency of around 70 beats/min, a normal sinoatrial pacemaker is present. However, the rate of QRS complexes denoting ventricular activation is only about 42 beats/min and there is no coordination of these events with P waves. This indicates that electrical activities in atria and ventricles are independent of each other.

17.D. In general, ectopic pacemakers in the atrioventricular region or the bundle of His discharge at frequencies of 50–60 beats/min. A lower ventricular frequency suggests that the pacemaker is located in a bundle branch or the myocardium. This is supported by the notched R wave, which indicates a timing mismatch in delivery of action potentials to the two ventricles. In this case, a myocardial pacemaker can be excluded on two grounds. First, the absolute discharge frequency of myocardial ectopic foci is only around 15–30 beats/min, rather than the 42 beats/min seen here. Second, an action potential originating from a site within the myocardium would travel much more slowly through the ventricular syncytium than would one that entered several myocardial sites simultaneously via the Purkinje system. Therefore, the QRS complex would be at least twice as long as normal. The QRS complex in the present case is only moderately prolonged above the normal 60–80 ms.

18.C. The normal oncotic pressure of plasma is 26–28 mmHg, so intracapillary hydrostatic pressure must exceed this value before net extravasation of water occurs. Because pulmonary venous vascular resistance is very low, intravascular pressure falls by only around 2 mmHg between pulmonary capillaries and left atrium. A left atrial pressure of 25 mmHg will therefore result in 27 mmHg in the capillaries.

These values are useful for the purposes of illustrating the results of an acute rise in left atrial pressure, such as might result from a myocardial infarct and which can lead to fatal oedema within an hour. By contrast, if there is progressive chronic elevation in left atrial pressure there is usually a considerable degree of compensation due to improved lymphatic drainage of the lung. In consequence, patients in Mr O'R.'s situation are often able to survive with left atrial and pulmonary capillary pressures considerably higher than those that can be calculated to cause oedema.

19.B. The thiazides are widely used agents that have only moderate diuretic effects because they selectively inhibit sodium reabsorption in the distal convoluted tubule, where less than 10% of total sodium reabsorption occurs. Thiazides have the side-effect of causing potassium depletion, secondary to the increased amount of sodium that passes through the distal tubule. Other classes of diuretic include the acetazolamides, which act through inhibition of carbonic anhydrase and so tend to disturb acid–base balance, and the inhibitors of sodium–potassium–chloride symport, such as furosemide, that act in the loop of Henle.

20.B. Warfarin is a coumarin-type anticoagulant that blocks the binding site for vitamin K on its hepatic apoenzyme. This prevents formation of prothrombin and of various clotting factors further upstream (factors VII, IX, X, protein C). The effect of warfarin is enhanced by many antibiotics because these deplete the normal colonic microflora that represent the body's main source of vitamin K. Haemophilia, incidently, is due to a selective defect in factor VIII production.

CASE REVIEW

Stenotic damage to the aortic valve is the single most common valvular defect. It originates in inflammatory thickening of the valve leaflets, which leads to local fibrosis and lipoprotein deposition. The lipoprotein subsequently calcifies, reducing the leaflet flexibility that is needed for normal valve opening but usually not impairing its capacity to shut. The majority of cases of adult aortic stenosis occur in elderly men, especially those of Caucasian origins. Because lipoprotein is involved in lesion formation, it is likely that high plasma levels of low-density lipoprotein contribute to the stenotic process in this patient group. A second population at risk is children and adolescents, in whom valvular inflammation is an autoimmune consequence of systemic infection by group A haemolytic streptococci (*rheumatic fever*). With the availability of prompt antibiotic cover, rheumatic fever is now rare in Western societies, but it continues to be a common event in developing countries.

Aortic stenosis illustrates dramatically the interrelation between cardiac structure and function, and many aspects of the clinical presentation can be deduced from a knowledge of the normal cardiac cycle. For instance, the second heart sound is often softer than normal, because the aortic valve leaflets do not move as far as usual when they shut at the end of systole. In the normal heart, right side ejection usually finishes slightly later than that from the left side because of the relatively small amount of right ventricular muscle, leading to the pulmonary component of the second heart sound being slightly later than the aortic component (splitting). The sequence of this splitting is reversed in aortic stenosis because of prolonged ejection through the narrowed aortic orifice (reversed splitting). Another instance of the underlying cardiovascular logic is the shape of the first heart sound. In the normal heart, the loudest part of this is the earliest segment corresponding to the time of atrioventricular valve shutting, and the intensity of the sound tapers off rapidly during isovolumetric contraction. In the heart with a stenotic aortic valve, the initial segment of the first sound is less intense than normal because the heart is distended and therefore vibrates less. The intensity then rises progressively, peaking during mid-ejection.

Aortic stenosis also illustrates the fact that clinical reality can be counter-intuitive in terms of the underlying physiological events. For example, it seems logical that increased severity of stenosis should increase the amount of systolic turbulence and hence the loudness of the systolic murmur. In fact, extremely severe stenosis is often associated with a less intense murmur because of the very small volume of blood that is ejected. Also, despite the apparent dependence of cardiac output and blood pressure control on normal ventricular outflow, most individuals with aortic stenosis have no symptoms even during exercise until a late stage of the disease, because of compensating cardiac hypertrophy. After this stage has been reached, however, the risk of fatal myocardial ischaemia or pulmonary oedema rises dramatically and life expectancy is only 2–3 years without surgical intervention.

For the sake of illustration, investigation of the patient in this case relied on left heart catheterization to confirm the diagnosis. Nowadays, equivalent information on left mechanical function can usually be obtained non-invasively by echocardiography, and left heart catheterization is no longer so widely used as it carries a finite risk of adverse events. However, arterial catheterization is still an essential part of preoperative assessment, as it is needed for angiographic evaluation of the coronary circulation.

Several types of artificial valves are available, some working on a ball-and-cage design such as was used here and some based on hinged tilting discs. An alternative approach is to implant a real valve taken from a pig or ox or, occasionally, of human origin. The advantage of these tissue prostheses is that they do not stimulate thrombus formation: with a mechanical valve, permanent anticoagulant cover is needed. On the other hand, the mechanical valves are robust and long-lived, while tissue implants usually deteriorate in less than 10 years. They are therefore contraindicated for use in young patients.

KEY POINTS

- Aortic stenosis is the most common single valve cardiac lesion, occurring most frequently in children and elderly men.
- The usual cause is inflammatory fibrosis of the valve leaflets, with subsequent calcium deposition.
- This process may be accelerated in the presence of hyperlipidaemia.

- The characteristic symptoms of aortic stenosis reflect reduced cardiac reserve during situations that require elevated cardiac output – angina, breathlessness and syncope.
- Once stenosis is severe enough to cause these symptoms, life expectancy is only 2–3 years unless surgical valve replacement is undertaken.

ADDITIONAL READING

Boudoulas H (2003) Etiology of valvular heart disease. *Expert Review of Cardiovascular Therapy* 1: 523–32.

Demer LL (2001) Cholesterol in vascular and valvular calcification. *Circulation* 104: 1881–3.

Edhouse J, Thakur RK & Khalil JM (2002) ABC of clinical electrocardiography: conditions affecting the left side of the heart. *British Medical Journal* 324: 1264–7.

Goldsmith I, Turpie AGG & Lip GYH (2002) ABC of antithrombotic therapy: valvar heart disease and prosthetic heart valves. *British Medical Journal* 325: 1228–31.

McCann GP & Hillis WS (2004) Surgery in asymptomatic aortic stenosis. *British Medical Journal* 328: 63–4.

Wu, WC, Ireland LA & Sadaniantz A (2004) Evaluation of aortic valve disorders using stress echocardiography. *Echocardiography* 21: 459–66.

Tiredness and failure to mature

CASE AND MCQS

Case introduction

Lisa N. is a 16-year-old girl who has been brought to your office by her parents. They are concerned that she is very skinny, has not gone through puberty, and is always tired. They state that she eats well, appears to be happy and used to get along very well with her friends and classmates. More recently, however, the others all appear to be much more grown up and Lisa has become withdrawn.

On examination, Lisa is 160 cm (5 ft 3 in) in height, weighs 40 kg (88 lb) and appears physically underdeveloped for 16 years old.

Her blood pressure is 100/65 mmHg, her pulse rate is 76 beats/min. She looks pale and her conjunctivae and tongue are pale. She has a systolic murmur, maximal at the apex. Her nails show signs of increased mooning and there are also white lines higher up in the nails, suggesting some episodic occurrence.

You order a full blood examination and plasma biochemistry and ask her to return in one week's time.

Normal ranges of values expected for a blood count are:

Haemoglobin (Hb)	11.5 – 16.5 g/dl
Haematocrit (Hct)	35–48%
Red cell count	3.5–5.4 × 10^{12}/l
Mean red cell volume (MCV)	82 – 95 fl
Mean red cell Hb concentration (MCHC)	320–360 g/l

Table 10.1 lists five sets of data obtained from different patients.

Table 10.1 Five sets of blood count values for different patients

	Haemoglobin (g/dl)	Haematocrit (%)	Red cell count (× 10^{12}/l)	Mean red cell volume (fl)	Mean red cell haemoglobin concentration (g/l)
A	10.0	34	5.1	66	294
B	12.0	42	4.0	84	360
C	14.6	43	4.9	88	340
D	16.8	46	5.6	83	350
E	11.0	36	3.5	103	306

Q1 Which of the results in Table 10.1 is most likely in a normal 16-year-old female?

Q2 Which of the results in Table 10.1 is most likely in a normal 16-year-old male?

Q3 Which of the results in Table 10.1 is most likely in a person with thalassaemia?

Q4 Which of the results in Table 10.1 is most likely in a person with iron-deficiency anaemia?

Q5 Which of the results in Table 10.1 is most likely in a person with vitamin B_{12} deficiency?

You see Lisa again one week later. Her haematological values are:

Haemoglobin	9.5 g/dl
Haematocrit	32%
Red cell count	5.0×10^{12}/l
Mean corpuscular volume	64 fl
Mean corpuscular haemoglobin concentration	300 g/l

Her plasma biochemistry is as follows:

Sodium	135 mmol/l
Potassium	3.5 mmol/l
Creatinine	0.06 mmol/l
Urea	2.4 mmol/l
Calcium	2.11 mmol/l
Glucose	3.6 mmol/l
Cholesterol	3.0 mmol/l
Total protein	65 g/l
Albumin	35 g/l

At this time you ask her in more detail about her eating. She states that most of the time she eats well and has no problems. But episodically, about once per month, she does develop some abdominal pains and with this, diarrhoea. Her faeces at that time appear to be relatively pale and are offensive in smell. On other occasions she develops watery diarrhoea. This has been going on for the last 4–5 years and appears to be exacerbated when she eats fast food with her friends.

At home she rarely eats bread or cereal as she feels these may upset her, and her parents tell her that she is picky about her food. She also states that her hair is not shiny and that she does not like its appearance. You ask her does she vomit after a meal and she states definitely no.

Q6 How would you determine if Lisa's problem is due to psychological causes or to an organic lesion? What is your own belief about its basis at this time?

You perform some investigations of Lisa's gastrointestinal tract function and obtain the following results:
- 24-hour faecal fat is three-fold above the upper limit of normal (*steatorrhoea*)
- Xylose absorption (a marker of hexosesugar absorption) is impaired.

You also order plasma levels of a number of other substances, but will have to wait for these results.

Q7 The elevation of faecal fats to three times the normal level could be due to:

A. lack of bile acids in the intestine
B. lack of pancreatic lipase
C. impaired intestinal mucosal function
D. any of A, B or C
E. either B and C

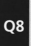

Q8 Lack of bile acids in the intestine leads directly or indirectly to malabsorption of many substances. Which of the following substances is *not* malabsorbed in the absence of bile salts?

A. vitamin D
B. vitamin K
C. complex lipids
D. vitamin B_{12}
E. calcium

Q9 In relation to the absorption of carbohydrates, which of the following statements is *not* correct?

A. maltase and lactase are disaccharidases
B. disaccharidases are intestinal membrane enzymes
C. absorption of glucose depends on a sodium–glucose co-transport system
D. hexosesugars all use a common co-transporter for absorption
E. alpha-amylase breaks down starches to limit dextrins

Q10 In relation to the digestion of proteins, which of the following statements is *not* correct?

A. trypsinogen is activated by enterokinase
B. trypsinogen is activated by trypsin
C. typsinogen is activated by alkaline pH
D. trypsinogen is not activated in the pancreas
E. trypsinogen is an endopeptidase

At this time it is worth considering what you have found and where you go from here. Lisa has:
- Anaemia – but what is the cause?
- Low albumin, low urea – indicates lack of protein in the body due to failure of intake or poor absorption.
- Low glucose, abnormal xylose absorption – indicates abnormal carbohydrate absorption.
- High faecal fats – indicates poor fat digestion and/or absorption.
- Low plasma calcium level.

Q11 What is the most likely cause of the above abnormal group of results?

A. psychosomatic anorexia nervosa
B. failure of secretion of pancreatic enzymes
C. lack of bile acids and bile salts
D. poor intestinal absorption of nutrients
E. deficient intake of nutrients

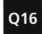

Q12 Which of the following may be contributing to Lisa's anaemia?

A. low plasma iron
B. low vitamin B$_{12}$
C. low folic acid
D. either B and C
E. any of A, B, and C

Iron is essential for haemoglobin formation and for activity of the cytochrome system.

Q13 Which of the following factors related to iron metabolism is *not* correct?

A. iron is more readily absorbed when it is associated with haemoglobin
B. iron absorption takes place mainly in the duodenum
C. ferrous salts are absorbed more readily than ferric salts
D. excess absorbed iron is excreted by the kidney
E. women need more iron in the diet than men

Q14 Which of the following statements related to iron absorption or transport is *not* correct?

A. transferrin is the transport protein for iron
B. ferritin is the storage form of iron
C. plasma transferrin levels are decreased in iron deficiency
D. ferritin levels are decreased in iron deficiency
E. ferritin in intestinal cells prevents excessive absorption of iron

Q15 Lisa reports that she has watery stools (diarrhoea) on occasions. Which of the following is most likely to be causing this diarrhoea?

A. excessive crypt secretion of chloride and water
B. increased osmolality in the intestinal lumen
C. poor absorption of sodium by the intestinal mucosa
D. none of the above
E. all of A, B and C

Q16 In the normal control of sodium and water absorption by the intestine, which of the following is *not* correct?

A. increased intracellular cyclic AMP stimulates crypt cell secretion of chloride and water
B. increased intracellular cyclic AMP inhibits mucosal cell reabsorption of sodium and water
C. increased intracellular cyclic GMP inhibits mucosal cell reabsorption of sodium and water
D. increased cytoplasmic ionized calcium increases mucosal cell reabsorption of Na$^+$ and water
E. cholera toxin increases cyclic AMP levels in mucosal cells

Q17 If a person had impaired function of the terminal ileum, the absorption of which of the following substances would *not* be impaired?

A. vitamin B$_{12}$
B. iron
C. calcium
D. vitamin D
E. vitamin K

The results of the other blood investigations that you ordered are returned. The values are (normal values in brackets):

Serum iron	5 µmol/l (5.0–30)
Total serum iron-binding capacity	60 µmol/l (45–73)
Serum iron saturation	8% (25–45)
Ferritin	48 µg/l (11–307)
Vitamin B$_{12}$	120 µg/ml (150–700)
Folate	3.0 µg/l (5–20)

These values indicate severe iron depletion, moderate B$_{12}$ depletion and low folic acid. The red cell indices indicate a complex picture with features of microcytic hypochromic anaemia (suggesting iron deficiency) but also some abnormal cell forms (suggesting deficiencies of B$_{12}$ and folic acid).

Considering all the possibilities, you conclude that this is a case of generalized malabsorption by the intestine, rather than a specific defect. Your decision is based on the fact that absorption of fats, carbohydrates, protein, iron, vitamin B$_{12}$ and calcium are all impaired. This indicates a generalized mucosal defect rather than any specific enzymatic defect.

You perform a biopsy of the intestinal mucosa which shows a flattened epithelium, a paucity of villi, and inflammatory cells in the submucosa. This allows you to make a final diagnosis of gluten sensitivity (*coeliac disease*).

You prescribe a diet that does not contain wheat products, since this is the principal source of gluten. On this diet Lisa improves rapidly but notes that if she eats products containing wheat, she develops acute gastrointestinal symptoms. She learns to avoid wheat products.

MCQ ANSWERS AND FEEDBACK

1.C; 2.D. Both sets of values for these are in the normal range but, in general, males have a greater number of red cells than females, resulting in a higher haematocrit and haemoglobin.

3A. Thalassaemia is due to abnormal haemoglobins and is an inherited disease relatively common in Mediterranean people. In its mild form it causes relatively few problems. The red cell indices are similar to those found in a person with iron-deficiency anaemia, but plasma iron levels are markedly different.

4.A. This is a *hypochromic* (low cell Hb concentration) and *microcytic* (low cell volume) anaemia and is a typical pattern resulting from iron depletion.

5.E. This is a *macrocytic* (large cell volume) anaemia. A similar pattern would be seen with both vitamin B_{12} and folic acid deficiency.

6. It is very difficult to determine if the situation has a psychological cause (for example, anorexia nervosa). Anorexia nervosa may be difficult to diagnose and even more difficult to treat. However, in this patient the story of diarrhoea and the presence of anaemia leads one to suspect an organic cause.

7.E. Lack of bile acids leads to a slowing of the digestion of fats and malabsorption of complex lipids but rarely to frank steatorrhoea. However, lack of pancreatic lipase and poor mucosal function can both lead to this degree of steatorrhoea.

8.D. Lack of bile acids leads to malabsorption of vitamins D, K and A, and other complex lipids. Poor levels of vitamin D lead to calcium malabsorption. B_{12} absorption, however, is not affected.

9.D. Alpha-amylase breaks down starches to limit dextrins, which are broken down further to disaccharides by dextrinase, and to monosaccharides by specific disaccharidases (particularly maltase, sucrase, lactase), which are intestinal membrane enzymes. The hexosesugars, except for fructose, use the same sodium-dependent co-transporter but fructose (a hexosesugar) is absorbed by diffusion using its own carrier.

10.C. Trypsinogen is the inactive precursor of trypsin. It is activated by enterokinase, an enzyme in the duodenum, and then trypsin can self-activate trypsinogen and other proteolytic enzyme precursors. It is not activated by a high pH and is not activated in the pancreas. Trypsin is an endopeptidase (that is, it breaks down bonds inside the peptide sequence).

11.D. There are multiple defects present. The only answer listed that can explain all of these defects is poor mucosal absorption. Lack of secretion of pancreatic enzymes would produce steatorrhoea and impaired protein digestion, but xylose absorption would be normal.

12.E. With a mucosal defect, absorption of all three substances and also of protein would be impaired, and all of these may contribute to the anaemia.

13.D. The intestine regulates the iron content of the body by controlling absorption. The kidney excretes very little iron in normal circumstances, but can be made to excrete more by using chelating compounds. The mechanism of control of iron absorption is indicated in Fig. 10.1. When iron is in excess it is bound to ferritin in the intestinal mucosal cell, which is then sloughed off and lost in the faeces.

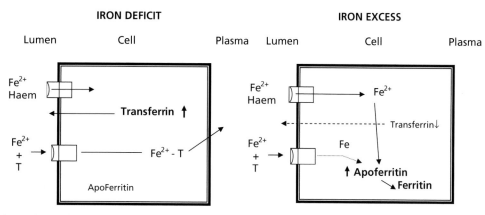

Fig. 10.1 Mechanisms of iron absorption.

14.C. In iron deficiency, the production of transferrin increases in the liver and in the intestinal cells (Fig. 10.1). Transferrin is secreted into the bowel and binds to iron, which can then cross the cell membrane and go through the cell and be transported to the tissues to be used. Ferritin is the storage form of iron and, when iron levels are high, production of the apoprotein is increased in the body and in the intestinal cells. In the intestinal cells this binds the iron that enters the cell, thereby preventing its absorption.

15.E. The crypt cells secrete chloride and water follows. In gluten sensitivity there is usually increased proliferation of crypt cells but the problem is the cells do not migrate along the villi, which are reduced in number and size. Absorption of water follows the absorption of sodium by mucosal cells in the villi, so water uptake is defective when there is poor mucosal function. The poor absorption of amino acids, hexosesugars and fatty acids mean that there are more osmolytes in the lumen that will hold water. Thus A, B and C all contribute to the diarrhoea.

16.D. The secretion of chloride by crypt cells and the inhibition of sodium absorption by the villi cells are both controlled by cyclic AMP levels. Increased cyclic AMP causes increased secretion of chloride and increased cyclic AMP inhibits sodium absorption. Cyclic GMP, which may be increased by toxins from various bacteria such as *Escherichia coli*, inhibits sodium absorption. Increased cytoplasmic calcium also inhibits sodium absorption. Cholera toxins cause profuse watery diarrhoea by increasing cellular cyclic AMP levels.

17.B. Vitamins B_{12}, D and K are all absorbed in the terminal ileum and so their absorption is impaired. Calcium absorption is also impaired due to lack of vitamin D. Iron is absorbed predominantly in the duodenum and would not be affected in a person with disease or absence of the terminal ileum.

CASE REVIEW

Anaemia can result from a number of causes. There may be increased rate of destruction of red cells which exceeds the generative capacity of the bone marrow, thus resulting in low haemoglobin. The most common basis for this is inheritance of an abnormal form of haemoglobin which reduces red cell half-life and gives a typical morphological appearance to the red cells. This inherited defect of thalassaemia is common in people of Mediterranean descent. Other abnormal haemoglobins occur in other parts of the world but are not as common.

A second cause is poor red cell formation. The most common reason is lack of vitamin B_{12} and/or folic acid. These substances are essential for maturation of all cells, but abnormalities in the red cells with anaemia usually result first. Once again, this type of anaemia is characterized by a typical morphology of the red cells, with macrocytosis. Vitamin B_{12} deficiency can result from a lack of vitamin B_{12} in the diet, lack of intrinsic factor produced in the oxyntic cell of the gastric gland, and poor absorption of the complex of vitamin B_{12} and intrinsic factor which takes place in the terminal ileum. Folic acid can result from a lack in the diet or a failure of absorption. Poor red cell formation can also result from severe protein deficiency.

The most common cause of anaemia is a lack o s haemoglobin is not formed adequately and is not properly incorporated into the cells. A typical pattern of microcytic, hypochromic anaemia results. Iron deficiency most often results from blood loss. The absorption of iron and the amount stored in the body are regulated by the bowel, as the kidney has little excretory capacity (Fig. 10.1).

The absorption balances iron loss caused by blood loss, shedding of skin, etc. If iron absorption is not controlled, iron overload can result, leading to *haemochromatosis*. Iron deficiency can also result from malabsorption of iron or lack of absorbable iron in the diet. It is more common in women than in men because they lose blood at menstruation and lose additional iron during pregnancy and lactation. In Lisa's case iron, folic acid and vitamin B_{12} were all poorly absorbed but her anaemia, as indicated from the morphology, was mainly due to iron deficiency.

Failure of digestion and malabsorption may be generalized or specific. Thus, bile salt lack leads to malabsorption of complex lipids such as the fat-soluble vitamins A, D and K, with subsequent effects on absorption of calcium due to lack of vitamin D (Fig. 10.2). Specific enzymatic defects such as absence of lactase lead to accumulation of lactose in the intestinal lumen and osmotic diarrhoea. The pancreas produces a large number of enzymes involved in the digestion of carbohydrates, proteins and fats. If there are no pancreatic enzymes, there are sufficient other enzymes in the gastrointestinal tract to allow carbohydrate digestion and absorption to take place. A similar situation applies to protein digestion, although here the reserve is not quite so robust and problems in breakdown may occur.

The primary problem in pancreatic insufficiency is that there is no pancreatic lipase. If pancreatic lipase is not present, triglycerides are not broken down or absorbed and this leads to steatorrhoea (fatty stools). Fat-soluble vitamins are also not well absorbed as they stay dissolved in the fat in the stool. Lisa had malabsorption of iron, fats, vitamin B_{12}, folic acid,

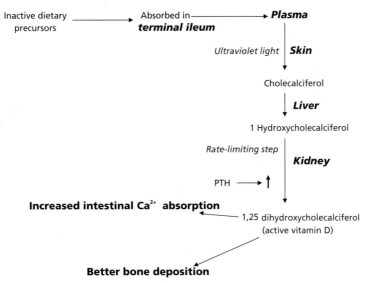

Fig. 10.2 Role of vitamin D in calcium handling by the body.

carbohydrates, proteins and calcium. This multiplicity of defects can only occur with a generalized gastrointestinal mucosal impairment.

The particular cause in Lisa's case, and a common cause around the world, is sensitivity to the gluten protein in wheat. Normally the mucosa has a convoluted structure with numerous villi (Fig. 10.3). In gluten-sensitive individuals, the gluten exerts a toxic effect on the villar epithelium. As a result, there is increased proliferation of crypt cells but the villi are immature and small, with insufficient membrane-bound enzymes to allow digestion to be completed and insufficient transporters, leading to malabsorption of all compounds. If a person is not exposed to gluten this problem can resolve. The disease can present in many forms, from generalized failure of absorption to specific defects where malabsorption of only one nutrient is apparent, although the capacity is markedly reduced for most substances if the digestion and absorption of these substances is measured.

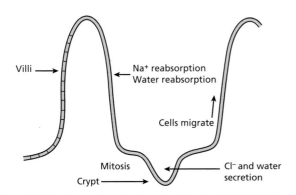
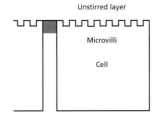
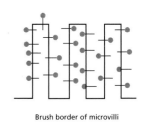

Fig. 10.3 Sodium and water handling by the intestinal villus.

ADDITIONAL READING

Farrell RT & Kelly CP (2002) Coeliac sprue. *New England Journal of Medicine* 346: 180–7.

Fasano A, Berti I & Gerarduzzi T (2003) Prevalence of coeliac disease in at risk and the not at risk group in the United States. *Archives of Internal Medicine* 163: 286–97.

Johnson LR (2001) *Gastrointestinal Physiology*, 6th edition. Mosby, St Louis.

Mäki M & Collin, P. (1997) Coeliac disease. *Lancet* 349: 1755–9.

Souhami RL & Moxham T (2002) *Textbook of Medicine*, 4th edition. Churchill Livingstone, London.

A stab wound to the chest

CASE AND MCQS

Case introduction

It is a summer night and the outside temperature is 28°C. At around 23.00 hours, a 32-year-old computer programmer (B.C.) is brought into hospital with a stab wound to the left side of his anterior chest wall. The wound had been inflicted outside a bar after an argument and altercation approximately 30 minutes earlier.

On the way to hospital an intravenous catheter had been inserted and a slow saline drip established. On arrival he is quiet but is complaining strongly of pain on his left side.

The ambulance crew found the weapon lying next to Mr C. and have brought it to hospital. It is a pocket-knife with a 10-cm non-serrated blade.

Examination shows an awake but pale and restless man breathing rapidly and shallowly, with a stab wound at the level of the left nipple. His heart rate is 132 beats/min, his blood pressure is 100/80 mmHg and his respiration rate is 32 breaths/min. His radial and groin pulses are bilaterally thin and thready. His legs are cool and pale.

Q1 In relation to his vital signs:

A. heart rate and blood pressure are normal
B. respiratory rate is within normal resting limits
C. peripheral perfusion appears normal
D. none of A, B and C
E. all of A, B and C

Chest examination with a stethoscope reveals that he has decreased breath sounds on the left side. His arterial oxygen saturation, taken with an ear oximeter, is 75%.

Think about what major organs might be involved. Then think about the immediate actions that are needed.

Q2 What are the major organs likely to be affected?

Q3 What are the major priorities now? Make a list.

In relation to the mechanics of resting breathing, the respiratory muscles, thoracic wall and diaphragm operate on the lungs to induce a regular expansion of the lung (inspiration) followed by their relaxation and expiration of air. Normally the lungs fill the major part of the thoracic space and they and the inner chest wall are surrounded by two layers of a membrane that enclose a potential space.

Q4 The potential space between the lungs and thoracic wall is:

A. the alveolar space
B. the mediastinal space
C. the pleural space
D. the anatomical dead space
E. none of the above

Q5 Pressure within this potential space during quiet respiration:

A. is always negative relative to atmospheric pressure
B. is always positive relative to atmospheric pressure
C. changes from negative to positive depending on the phase of respiration
D. is equal to atmospheric pressure except during expiration
E. is equal to atmospheric pressure at all times

Q6 The absolute value of this pressure is determined by:

A. diaphragmatic activity
B. elasticity of the lungs
C. rigidity of the chest wall
D. thoracic volume
E. all of the above

Q7 During inspiration, alveolar pressure:

A. is greater than atmospheric pressure
B. is less than atmospheric pressure
C. remains identical to atmospheric pressure
D. first rises above and then falls below atmospheric pressure
E. first falls below and then rises above atmospheric pressure

Thus, during inspiration, elastic recoil opposes inflation of the lungs and intrapleural pressure has to be more negative to achieve inflation. Conversely, during expiration where elastic recoil assists expiratory air flow, intrapleural pressure becomes less negative. During both inspiration and expiration, airway resistance opposes the change in lung volume.

Q8 An increase in airway resistance will result, during inspiration, in:

A. intrapleural pressure becoming less negative
B. intrapleural pressure becoming more negative
C. intrapleural pressure being unchanged
D. either B or C depending on the absolute lung volume
E. none of the above

If there is a perforation of the thoracic wall or the lung, the intrapleural pressure becomes atmospheric and the lung collapses, leaving an air-filled pleural space (pneumothorax). If the opening remains open, air moves in and out as the patient breathes.

Q9 If the thoracic cavity is opened to the atmosphere, the lung collapses because of:

A. the elastic recoil of the lung tissue
B. compression of the lung by air in the thorax
C. reduced resistance to airflow
D. descent of the diaphragm
E. all of the above

If, for some reason, the opening into the thoracic cage is then closed, for example by a flap of muscle or skin that falls across the opening, this has further consequences for respiration.

Q10 If the opening is closed, pressure in the pleural space will:

A. remain the same as atmospheric
B. decrease to a stable negative value
C. increase and decrease in parallel with respiratory movements
D. be atmospheric or supra-atmospheric depending on the phase of respiration
E. both C and D above

As described in the answer to Question 10, an intermittent tension pneumothorax can result in a progressive rise in intrathoracic pressure.

Q11 Elevation of intrathoracic pressure will preferentially reduce:

A. gas transfer in the lung
B. blood flow in great veins
C. movement of the diaphragm
D. aortic blood flow
E. B and C above

At this stage it should be noted that the impact of a unilateral pneumothorax in humans is largely restricted to the affected side. This is because of the relatively firm support provided by the mediastinum.

Let us now look at the effects of the collapsed lung on gas transport. Essentially, this will result in a veno-arterial shunt.

Q12 Veno-arterial shunting in a collapsed lung is the result of:

A. passage of pulmonary capillary blood past non-ventilated alveoli
B. reduced ventilation of the collapsed tissue
C. altered ventilation/perfusion ratio in the collapsed tissue
D. all of A, B and C above
E. none of the above

What is to be done for B.C. now? It is important to ensure that he is properly oxygenated so oxygen should be administered through a facemask; this should improve his O_2 saturation, which needs to be monitored. The unilateral breath sounds should be investigated and the wound probed to open the aperture. Inward and outward air movement during respiration can usually be heard.

A chest X-ray would help to confirm the existence of a pneumothorax. This would appear as a deviation of the mediastinum and heart to the opposite side together with a clear image of collapsed lung tissue on the affected side.

You insert a chest drain. After a short time blood appears and over 30 minutes approximately 500 ml accumulates, indicating that there is bleeding within the thorax.

This conclusion is confirmed by Mr C.'s condition, which is now beginning to deteriorate. His vital signs are now:

Heart rate	98 beats/min
Blood pressure	100/60 mmHg
Respiratory rate	25 breaths/min

His skin is still pale and his peripheral pulse is still thin and thready.

Before looking at the next steps we can usefully examine some of the body's responses to blood loss. Although 500 ml blood has been collected, this may not be an accurate reflection of how much haemorrhage has actually occurred and comparing known responses to specific degrees of blood loss with Mr C.'s vital signs will help in estimating the true volume that has been lost.

Q13 **In an individual with a blood volume of 5 litres, loss of 500 ml blood will cause:**

A. low pulse pressure and a raised heart rate
B. low systolic pressure and raised heart rate
C. low diastolic blood pressure and raised heart rate
D. all of the above
E. none of the above

The reflex responses that are activated by blood loss involve changes in the behaviour of both low-pressure (atrial) and high-pressure (carotid sinus and aortic arch) baroreceptors. How does this behaviour change and what is the efferent limb of some of the reflex changes that result?

Q14 **In relation to innervation of the blood vessels, blood loss results in:**

A. increased baroreceptor firing and a reflex increase in sympathetic firing
B. decreased baroreceptor firing and a reflex decrease in sympathetic firing
C. decreased baroreceptor firing and a reflex increase in sympathetic firing
D. increased baroreceptor firing and a reflex decrease in sympathetic firing
E. decreased baroreceptor firing and a reflex decrease in parasympathetic firing

---

Q15 **In relation to innervation of the heart, blood loss results in:**

A. an increase in vagal and an increase in sympathetic efferent impulses
B. a decrease in vagal and a decrease in sympathetic efferent impulses
C. a decrease in vagal and an increase in sympathetic efferent impulses
D. no change in vagal and sympathetic efferent impulses
E. no change in vagal and an increase in sympathetic efferent impulses

Note that, in addition to these changes, adrenaline may be secreted by the adrenal medulla and renin may be secreted from the kidney. These will also have the effect of stabilizing the blood pressure and restoring blood volume longer term. At the same time, there are alterations in the tissues resulting in an influx of extracellular fluid from the interstitial space into the circulating vascular space. These are a result of the reflex peripheral vasoconstriction.

Q16 **Movement of extracellular fluid into the capillaries as a result of peripheral vasoconstriction is due to:**

A. increased capillary blood pressure
B. increased plasma oncotic pressure
C. decreased plasma oncotic pressure
D. decreased capillary blood pressure
E. decreased venous pressure

In treatment of blood loss, the issues that need to be addressed are both the need to restore normal oxygen carriage capacity and the need to restore normal blood volume. If blood loss has not been so severe as to cause hypoxia, the issue of volume replacement could be handled by infusion of isotonic saline, or plasma, or a plasma substitute.

Q17 Isotonic saline is not a satisfactory fluid for replacing blood volume because it:

A. reduces plasma oncotic pressure
B. causes red cell lysis
C. dilutes the red cell mass
D. all of the above
E. both A and C above

Back to the patient. At this stage it is important to recognize that he is showing signs of both blood loss and respiratory insufficiency; measures are needed to stabilize him.

You need to stabilize his ventilation, and therefore insert an endotracheal tube and give him 100% oxygen to breathe, via a positive-pressure ventilator.

His high heart rate, low blood pressure, rapid respiration, pale skin, etc. are indicators that the blood loss from within the chest is having effects. You decide that he needs blood.

Q18 What type of blood can be given without waiting for a blood match?

A. Group A
B. Group B
C. Group O
D. Group AB
E. either Group A or Group B

You give him 500 ml (1 unit) of blood. His cardiovascular status improves after the blood infusion, with a rise in blood pressure to 110/70 mmHg and a fall in heart rate to 90 beats/min. His peripheral pulses are also firmer. However, a steady flow of blood still leaks from the chest.

It is obviously important to investigate the source of the internal bleeding. You ask for a chest X-ray to see if there is evidence of damage to other organs. This shows that the aorta has survived intact but it looks as though blood could be accumulating in the pericardial sac.

Mr C.'s heart rate and blood pressure begin to fall again and his peripheral pulses once again become thready, despite another unit of blood being infused.

Q19 List the potential effects of accumulation of blood in the pericardium.

It is decided that the best course of action is to do an exploratory thoracotomy. The patient is artificially ventilated and his chest opened. In addition to the collapsed left lung a small incision is found in the pericardium and in one of the pulmonary veins. These are sutured. The chest is then closed and a tube inserted into the left thoracic cavity, with the external end placed under water.

Q20 List the reasons why the external end of the chest drain should be placed under water.

After a few days Mr C.'s cardiovascular function and respiratory status are near normal. His chest drain is removed and he is discharged home.

MCQ ANSWERS AND FEEDBACK

1.D. Heart rate is higher than normal, pulse pressure is slightly low and respiration rate is higher than normal. The thready peripheral pulses and cool pale extremities are not consistent with normal peripheral blood flow on a warm night.

2. The major organs at risk are: lungs, heart, pericardium and great vessels.

3. The first priority is to determine the extent of damage. His respiration should be stabilized and controlled; the possibility of internal bleeding needs to be established and its extent identified and controlled. Is he already showing signs of significant blood loss? Think about his vital signs.

4.C. The pleural space or pleural cavity lies between the visceral and parietal pleura; it normally contains a thin layer of extracellular fluid that allows the lungs to slide inside the chest during the respiratory cycle.

5.A. Normally, intrapleural pressure is 3–12 mmHg (0.4–1.6 kPa) negative with respect to atmospheric pressure.

6.E. All contribute. Intrapleural pressure is negative because of the balance between two opposing forces, the tendency of the compliant lungs to collapse and the tendency of the more rigid thoracic wall to expand. The lungs are very compliant but are elastic and tend to collapse; the relatively rigid chest wall tends to oppose this collapse and the contraction of the diaphragm alters the volume of the chest and must therefore also affect intrapleural pressure. During relaxed expiration, the forces are at equilibrium and pressure is approximately 3–5 mmHg (0.4–0.7 kPa) negative. During inspiration, it becomes more negative (10–12 mmHg, 1.4–1.6 kPa) because of the increased intrathoracic volume.

7.B. When there is no airflow into or out of the lungs, alveolar pressure is atmospheric. When the ribcage chest enlarges and the diaphragm descends at the commencement of inspiration, alveolar pressure becomes negative and air passes into the lungs down the pressure gradient. As the lungs are very compliant, intrapleural pressure continues to become more negative until the inspiratory phase is complete.

8.B. The resistance to air flow means that the ribcage and inspiratory muscles must do more work and this is reflected in an increase in the negative intrapleural pressure.

9.A. All of the remainder are consequences of the elastic recoil.

10.E. If the opening closes for whatever reason, pressure will be affected by respiratory efforts and will rise and fall with inspiration and expiration respectively, at atmospheric to supra-atmospheric pressures. This is termed a tension pneumothorax. If the obstruction acts intermittently, for example acting like a 'flap valve' and opening only during inspiration, then increasing amounts of air can be sucked in. This will result in progressively increasing supra-atmospheric pressure in the thorax at all phases of the respiratory cycle.

11.B. The positive pleural pressure will affect venous return on the right and left sides of the heart since the transmural pressures across their walls will be diminished. Secondarily, in severe cases, cardiac output will be impeded.

12.D. Such a shunt in the lung indicates that some blood in the pulmonary capillaries is not being exposed to alveoli that are ventilated. That is, the *V/Q* relationship in the affected lung is disturbed. This will alter the movement of gases across the lung on the affected side but transport will be unaltered in the other lung. The net effect on blood gases will be serious.

13.E. Any fall in circulating blood volume will activate a series of reflexly evoked increases in heart rate and vascular resistance that have the intended effect of maintaining arterial blood pressure at its normal level. With falls in blood volume of 10–20% these reflex compensations cause elevated diastolic pressure and reduce systolic pressure, with mean pressure remaining constant. From this information, you can see that Mr C.'s low mean blood pressure suggests that he has lost more than 20% of his blood volume (Table 11.1).

14.C. Arterial baroreceptors sense the levels of blood pressure and the rate of change of pressure during the pulse wave. When blood pressure falls, the overall impulse traffic from the receptors declines and efferent sympathetic vasoconstrictor fibres to the vascular beds of skeletal muscles, splanchnic region and skin are excited to increase peripheral resistance and therefore blood pressure.

15.C. The reflex tachycardia that results from decreased firing of arterial baroreceptor fibres involves both inhibition of cardiac vagal activity and increased firing of sympathetic cardiac fibres.

16.D. Vasoconstriction in the peripheral arterioles and precapillary sphincters will result in lower capillary blood pressure. This will alter the balance of the Starling forces and interstitial fluid will move into the capillaries.

17.A. Remember that blood loss results in loss of cells and plasma, whereas infusion of saline adds fluid and ions only. Saline will disappear relatively quickly from the circulation into the interstitium because it dilutes the plasma proteins and so reduces plasma oncotic pressure. Red cell lysis will not occur because isotonic saline is by definition iso-osmotic with extracellular fluid. Addition of saline to the bloodstream will dilute the red cells but this will not further reduce oxygen-carrying capacity because the number of cells remains constant.

18.C. It is best to have the blood individually typed and to give that. But in an emergency when it is not possible to type rapidly, Group O (universal donor) should be given (Table 11.2). If you are uncertain, look up the basis of blood typing – the ABO system is the most common and important, as is the Rhesus system under certain conditions – think about these situations.

19. Leakage of blood into the pericardial cavity is termed *pericardial tamponade* and has important consequences even

Table 11.1 Summary of changes in blood pressure and heart rate associated with different degrees of blood volume reduction

Percentage blood volume reduction	Heart rate	Systolic blood pressure	Diastolic blood pressure	Pulse pressure
10% (500 ml)	Slight increase	No change	No change	No change
10–20% (500–1000 ml)	Progressive increase	Fall	Rise	Fall
>20% (1000 ml)	Progressive increase	Progressive fall	Progessive fall	Fall

The absolute volumes given are based on a typical normal blood volume of 5 litres.

Table 11.2 The ABO blood typing system

Blood type	RBC surface antigens present	Plasma antibodies present	Can donate blood to following	Can receive blood from following
A	A	Anti-B	A	A, O
B	B	Anti-A	B	B, O
AB	A + B	none	AB	A, B, AB, O (universal recipient)
O	none	Anti-A, Anti-B	A, B, AB, O (universal donor)	O

when the heart itself has not been damaged. The increased pressure in the cavity means that the transmural pressure across the cardiac chamber walls is reduced. This impairs both filling and contraction of atria and ventricles with the result that cardiac output and blood pressure are diminished.

20. While any obviously damaged vessels were tied, residual intrathoracic blood can continue to drain from the chest. Most importantly, the collapsed lung has been re-inflated by the artificial ventilation and placing the end of the tube about 5–7 cm under the water surface will restore a negative intrapleural pressure and enable the patient to be taken off the ventilator without his lung collapsing. Any residual gas in the intrapleural space will be progressively reabsorbed naturally (Fig. 11.1).

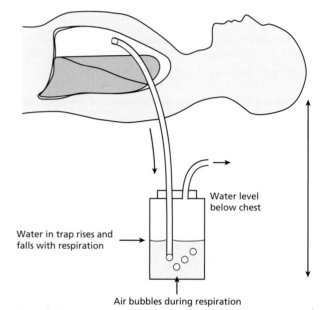

Water level below chest

Water in trap rises and falls with respiration

Air bubbles during respiration

Fig. 11.1 Arrangement of an intercostal chest drain to reduce a large pneumothorax. Correct placement of the drain can be judged by oscillation of the water level during respiration and continued removal of air from the thoracic cavity can be gauged by the production of bubbles. The water seal not only acts as a sterile one-way valve but also helps to keep drained body fluids from blocking the tube.

CASE REVIEW

The case illustrates the impact of a traumatic opening of the thorax on respiratory mechanics and consequential effects of this and bleeding on the cardiovascular system. Clearly any of the major tissues in the mid-chest area could have been damaged. If the wound had been lower in the ribcage then the possibility of additional damage to the diaphragm and upper abdominal organs would have had to be considered. In the present scenario it is obvious that the lungs are likely to be affected: other priorities for treatment are the extent of damage to great vessels or the heart and the extent of any bleeding.

Not all knife wounds to the chest would result in pericardial injury and great vessel injury but the important thing is to monitor the condition of the patient and try to assess which organs have been affected.

From a physiological point of view, the important aspects of this case relate to respiratory mechanics, ventilation/perfusion relationships in the lungs, blood typing and effects of blood loss. In practical terms, it is important first to establish control of ventilation and ensure that it is adequate, then tackle the bleeding and the potential cardiovascular consequences.

- Negative intrapleural pressure is essential in order for the lungs to change in volume during the respiratory cycle.
- Opening the pleural space to the atmosphere on one side of the chest reduces ventilatory volume and distorts ventilation/perfusion matching.
- In order to restore lung function after a traumatic pneumothorax it is necessary both to re-inflate the lung and to restore a negative intrapleural pressure.
- Penetrative wounds of the chest wall result predictably in both pneumothorax and intrathoracic haemorrhage.
- The proportion of blood loss that has resulted from haemorrhage can be estimated from the heart rate, the pulse pressure and the mean blood pressure, although compensatory mechanisms can maintain these variable within normal limits until the loss exceeds around 20% total blood volume.
- If the injury involves bleeding inside the pericardial cavity, then obstruction to cardiac filling by pericardial tamponade imposes a further limitation on circulatory function.

ADDITIONAL READING

Gutierrez G, Reins HD & Wulf-Gutierrez ME (2002) Haemorrhagic shock. *Critical Care* **8**: 373–81.

Mandal AK & Sanus M (2001) Penetrating chest wounds: 24 years experience. *World Journal of Surgery* **25**: 1145–9.

Miller AC & Harvey JE (1993) Guidelines for the management of spontaneous pneumothorax. *British Medical Journal* **307**: 114–16.

'I've gone yellow!'

CASE AND MCQS

Case introduction

A woman (R.F.) aged 45 presents to you and states that she has felt unwell for the past 10 days and is going yellow. You examine her and find that her conjunctivae are indeed yellow and that she is jaundiced.

Q1 Jaundice can result from all of the following *except*:

A. excessive bilirubin production by the liver
B. failure of conjugation of bilirubin
C. failure of uptake of bilirubin into liver cells
D. impaired secretion of bilirubin into the bile canaliculus
E. obstruction to the common bile duct

Q2 In a person with acute hepatocellular disease of the liver, which of the statements in Question 1 is the cause of the jaundice?

You obtain further information from the patient. She states that overall she has been in reasonable health but intermittently over the last 4–5 years she has had episodes of discomfort in the right hypochondrion. On two of these occasions there has been acute, colicky pain. These seem to be made worse by a fatty meal.

She was well until about 7–10 days ago, when she had what she thought was a viral infection and felt unwell. She has noticed that her urine has become darker than usual and 2 days ago friends commented that she looked yellow. She has not had much appetite over the last week and has had some discomfort over her liver.

On examination, all signs are normal except for jaundice and some tenderness in the right hypochondrion. This tenderness is not localized. The liver appears to be slightly enlarged and the liver edge is about 2 cm below the right costal margin.

You take blood for haematology and biochemistry.

Q3 Which of the following would explain the increased darkness of Ms F.'s urine?

A. increased urobilinogen
B. increased unconjugated bilirubin
C. increased bilirubin glucuronide
D. increased coproporphyrins
E. none of the above

Q4 Which one of the following tests is the most useful to distinguish obstructive from hepatocellular jaundice?

A. measurement of conjugated and unconjugated bilirubin
B. measurement of plasma levels of bile salts
C. measurement of coagulation profile
D. measurement of hepatic enzymes
E. measurement of lipoprotein profile

Q5 Which of the following statements regarding jaundice of different aetiology is *not* correct?

A. in haemolytic jaundice, conjugated bilirubin is elevated
B. in hepatocellular jaundice, conjugated bilirubin is elevated
C. in Gilbert's disease, conjugated bilirubin is elevated
D. in jaundice of prematurity, unconjugated bilirubin is elevated
E. in obstructive jaundice, conjugated bilirubin is elevated

Table 12.1 Five abnormal profiles for plasma markers of hepatic function

	Bilirubin	ALT	GGT	SAP	Coagulation time
A	72	450	500	200	Normal
B	57	600	500	130	↑↑
C	72	42	52	200	↑↑
D	44	26	24	60	Normal
E	32	26	24	60	↑↑

Table 12.1 shows several abnormal profiles for plasma markers of hepatic function. Normal enzyme values are:

Bilirubin	<18 µmol/l
Alanine aminotransferase (ALT)	<34 U/l
Gamma glutamyl transferase (GGT)	<38 U/l
Serum alkaline phosphatase (SAP)	<120 U/l

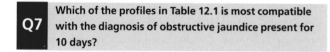

Q6 Which of the profiles in Table 12.1 is most compatible with the diagnosis of moderately severe hepatocellular jaundice?

Q7 Which of the profiles in Table 12.1 is most compatible with the diagnosis of obstructive jaundice present for 10 days?

Q8 Which of the profiles in Table 12.1 is most compatible with the diagnosis of haemolytic jaundice?

Q9 In moderately severe hepatocellular disease of one week duration, which of the following is *not* correct?

A. formation of active blood coagulation factors is impaired
B. the blood coagulation time is increased
C. synthesis of albumin is impaired
D. plasma transaminases are elevated
E. plasma albumin is reduced

Q10 Which of the following is useful to distinguish between hepatocellular and obstructive jaundice?

A. improved coagulation time with parenteral vitamin K
B. presence of urobilinogen in the urine
C. pale stools
D. both A and C
E. all of A, B and C

Q11 If a person has obstructive jaundice for 7–10 days, which of the following statements is *least* correct?

A. the stools will be pale
B. there will be steatorrhoea
C. the urine will be dark
D. there will be abnormal absorption of vitamin K
E. there will be abnormal absorption of vitamin D

The following results are returned from the biochemistry lab:

Urea	Normal
Creatinine	Normal
Electrolytes	Normal
Glucose	Normal
Protein	76 g/l
Albumin	42 g/l
Bilirubin	60 µmol/l
GGT	450 U/l
ALT	720 U/l
SAP	154 U/l
Coagulation time	Two times normal

Ms F.'s haemoglobin is normal, and red cell morphology and indices are all normal, but her stools are slightly paler than normal and her urine is dark.

You make a diagnosis of hepatocellular jaundice and you give an injection of vitamin K. You are, however, concerned by the elevation of SAP that was found and which is suggestive of obstructive jaundice. It would therefore be useful to visualize Ms F.'s intrahepatic ducts.

Q12 By what techniques could you determine if the intrahepatic ducts were distended and how could you objectively exclude obstructive jaundice?

Q13 In *acute* liver disease, elevation of plasma bilirubin is a prominent feature. In patients with *stable chronic* liver disease, a number of abnormalities may be seen but only one is invariably present. This is:

A. elevated liver enzymes
B. reduced plasma albumin
C. increased coagulation time
D. elevated bilirubin
E. salt and water retention

Q14 In chronic liver disease of moderate severity but in a quiescent phase (e.g. post-alcohol abuse but with current abstention), which one of the following is *least* likely to be present?

A. impaired plasma albumin synthesis
B. reduced plasma albumin concentration
C. elevated portal venous pressure
D. elevated plasma transaminases
E. reduced oestrogen metabolism

Q15 In chronic liver disease with sodium and water retention, which of the following is *least* likely to be present?

A. low blood pressure
B. reduced aldosterone secretion
C. reduced aldosterone metabolism
D. high portal venous pressure
E. normal blood volume

Imaging of Ms F.'s liver shows no distension of the intrahepatic ducts. She is placed under observation and after two weeks the jaundice begins to resolve and biochemical and liver function parameters all return to normal.

Immunological testing reveals that she has had hepatitis due to the hepatitis A virus.

MCQ ANSWERS AND FEEDBACK

1.A. Bilirubin is produced predominantly in the reticuloendothelial system. The spleen is a major site of breakdown of the haem part of haemoglobin to bilirubin. The bilirubin first formed is lipid-soluble and water-insoluble, and is transported to the liver loosely bound to albumin (Fig. 12.1). The bilirubin/albumin complex goes through the fenestrae of the sinusoids into the space of Disi and comes directly adjacent to the liver cell membrane. Bilirubin splits off the albumin and crosses this membrane by diffusion and/or by binding to a receptor. In the liver cell it is conjugated with glucuronide by an enzyme called glucuronyl-transferase to form water-soluble bilirubin glucuronide. This is secreted into the bile canaliculus and passes down the bile duct into the intestine. Jaundice can result from defects at any of these sites, labelled 1–3 in Fig. 12.1.

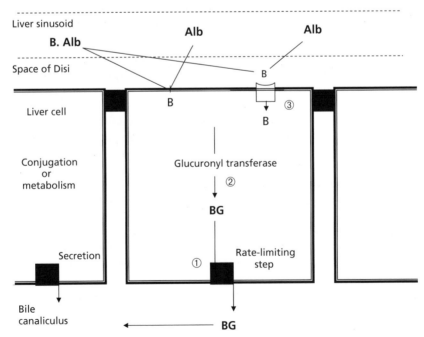

Fig. 12.1 Diagram of bilirubin processing in the liver, showing the sites of defects associated with (1) liver cell damage; (2) jaundice of prematurity; (3) Gilbert's disease. B, Bilirubin (lipid-soluble); Alb, albumin; BG, bilirubin glucuronide (water-soluble).

2.D. The rate-limiting step in the normal person is the transport (secretion) of bilirubin into the bile canaliculus (Fig. 12.1). Thus, if there is generalized damage to the liver cell, the process first affected is the secretion of bilirubin glucuronide, and bilirubin glucuronide (*conjugated* or *soluble* bilirubin) accumulates. If there is excessive production of bilirubin, both conjugated and unconjugated bilirubin accumulate.

3.C. Urobilinogen formed in the bowel by metabolism of bilirubin contributes to the normal colour of the urine, as also do uroporphyrins. In Ms F., however, the indications are that there is less bilirubin entering the bowel, as bilirubin has accumulated in the plasma. Unconjugated bilirubin is bound to albumin and thus does not enter the urine. The most likely cause of the dark urine, whether the jaundice is due to increased bilirubin production, to poor secretion of bilirubin or to bile duct obstruction, is the excretion of conjugated bilirubin in the urine.

4.D. There are abnormalities of all of these in jaundice due to each of the two causes. However, the best distinguishing test is the marked elevation of hepatic enzymes (AST, GGT) in hepatocellular disease and elevation of serum alkaline phosphatase (SAP) in obstructive disease.

5.C. Conjugated bilirubin is elevated in obstructive jaundice, hepatocellular jaundice and haemolytic jaundice. In jaundice of prematurity the enzyme glucuronyl-transferase is not present in adequate amounts, so unconjugated bilirubin is elevated and may cause toxic effects on the brain. In Gilbert's disease, the defect is either absence of receptors in the membrane causing poor uptake or a deficiency in conjugation. Thus unconjugated bilirubin is elevated. The extent of the elevation is small because some bilirubin can cross the membrane by diffusion and also because conjugation is not completely inhibited.

6.B. Moderately severe hepatocellular jaundice will cause marked elevation of liver enzymes and minor or no elevation of SAP. Impairment of coagulation will also be present.

7.C. Obstructive jaundice will cause elevation of SAP, minor changes in liver enzymes and a prolonged clotting time due to failure of absorption of vitamin K.

8.D. In haemolytic jaundice liver function is normal and therefore there are no increases in liver enzymes, SAP or clotting time unless there is accompanying severe anaemia, in which case minor changes may be seen secondary to impaired liver metabolism.

9.E. In moderately severe liver disease of one week duration there will be impaired synthesis of all proteins. Blood coagulation factor synthesis is impaired and as these factors have a short half-life of less than 3 days the clotting time is increased. Albumin synthesis is impaired but plasma albumin will have not yet fallen below normal, due to its long half-life. Oestrogen metabolism is impaired, as is that of aldosterone and corticosteroids, but over this period signs or symptoms are unlikely to be produced. Transaminases will be elevated.

10.E. Each of these is useful but not definitive. Thus in obstructive jaundice the stools are pale, there is no urobilinogen in the urine and the clotting time is prolonged. In obstructive jaundice, parenteral vitamin K improves clotting whilst there is no effect in hepatocellular disease.

11.B. The failure of bilirubin glucuronide to enter the bowel means the stools are pale and the urine is dark. The lack of bile acids in the bowel leads to malabsorption of complex lipids including vitamins D, K and A. Whilst digestion of fat may be slow due to a lack of bile acids, it does proceed and so steatorrhoea is uncommon.

12. Various imaging techniques can be used, all of which give useful information. They include ultrasound of the liver; computerized axial tomography (CAT scan) and visualization of the common bile duct with retrograde dye injection (*cholangiography*).

13.B. In patients with stable liver disease the liver enzymes are normal (or only mildly abnormal) because there is no acute damage to cells. The process that requires the greatest use of liver reserves is the production of albumin and the only defect present may be a low plasma albumin. Salt and water retention can occur but only when plasma albumin falls below a critical level.

14.D. Albumin synthesis is reduced and plasma albumin is low. Due to changes in the liver architecture the portal venous pressure will be high. Metabolism of steroid hormones including oestrogens is impaired and this may cause spider naevi to be present and, in males, feminization. In a quiescent phase, the liver enzymes may be normal or only slightly elevated.

15.B. The low plasma albumin activates forces in the body that lead to salt and water retention. This is mediated in part by activation of the renin–angiotensin–aldosterone system, so aldosterone secretion is increased. Plasma aldosterone also rises due to its impaired hepatic destruction. The portal venous pressure is high and this causes the retained fluid to be localized to the abdominal cavity. Measured circulating blood volume is normal or increased due to the increased volume in the portal system. However, functional circulating blood volume is likely to be reduced and therefore blood pressure may be low.

CASE REVIEW

Jaundice results from the accumulation of bilirubin in the body. This can be due to excessive production (*haemolytic jaundice*), failure of liver handling (*hepatocellular jaundice*) or failure of excretion (*obstructive jaundice*). There are other specific causes due to specific enzymatic or transport defects (Table 12.2). When bilirubin is formed in the reticuloendothelial system, particularly the spleen, it is in a lipid-soluble, water-insoluble form. It is carried loosely bound to albumin to the liver. It crosses the liver sinusoid into the space of Disi, adjacent to the liver cell membrane. The bilirubin may then bind to a membrane carrier and enter the cell, or dissolve in the lipid membrane and diffuse into the cell. Inside the cell, it is conjugated with glucuronide by the enzyme glucuronyl-transferase, making it water-soluble. It is then secreted into the bile canaliculus. This is the rate-limiting step (bottleneck) in the normal process of bilirubin handling.

The secreted bilirubin then flows into the bile duct system and may go to the gallbladder where it is concentrated up to 100-fold before being emptied by the common bile duct into the duodenum through the sphincter of Oddi. Bilirubin in the bowel is catalysed to various products including urobilinogen. Urobilinogen can be absorbed and is then excreted in the urine and provides a significant component of the normal urine colour. Bilirubin and its breakdown products (such as stercobilinogen) also give the normal brown colour to the faeces.

If plasma bilirubin is elevated, we can distinguish between the different forms of jaundice by the accompanying symptoms, signs and biochemical impairments although, in clinical medicine, it may not always be as easy as it appears in textbook cases.

In haemolytic jaundice, bilirubin production is increased (Table 12.3), leading to an increase in both unconjugated and conjugated bilirubin. This only occurs when the production is about 5–7 times normal, as the liver has a large reserve capacity. The defect may only appear when there is accompanying anaemia which reduces the liver's metabolic capacity. There will usually be no other abnormality of liver function measured biochemically. The faeces will be very dark due to increased bilirubin and its products in the faeces. The urine will be dark due to filtration and excretion of bilirubin glucuronide and there will be urobilinogen in the urine as there is bilirubin in the bowel.

In obstructive jaundice, liver function is normal but there will be accumulation of bile excretory products. Bilirubin is conjugated but it cannot exit the biliary system by the normal process and it leaks back into the plasma to be filtered and excreted by the kidney, leading to a dark urine. This is insufficient to maintain the plasma bilirubin at the normal level. The faeces will be pale due to absence of bilirubin and there will be no urobilinogen in the urine. Bile salts accumulate in the body and this can cause itching.

The other defects that exist relate to the absence of bile salts in the bowel. Absorption of vitamins A, D and K is impaired. There are reserves of vitamins A and D and no immediate problems result. However, there is no reserve of vitamin K and this is essential for a number of blood coagulation factors that are formed in the liver. These factors have a short half-life and rapidly become depleted, and coagulation problems may result. This can be measured as an increased coagulation time (often expressed in terms of the international normalization ratio, or INR) that returns to normal if an injection of vitamin

Table 12.2 Involvement of bilirubin in different types of hepatic disease

Structure	Function	Disease
Spleen	Bilirubin water-insoluble, formed from red cells	Haemolytic jaundice[a]
Portal blood	Carried bound to albumin	
Hepatic sinusoids	Freely permeable to albumin	Capillarization in chronic liver disease
Space of Disi	Space between sinusoid and liver cell	Fibrosis and thickness in chronic liver disease
Cell membranes	Permeable to bilirubin	Gilbert's disease[b]
	Carriers for bilirubin	
Hepatic cytoplasm	Glucuronyl-transferase (GT) makes bilirubin water-soluble	GT deficit in prematurity[b]
		Gilbert's disease[b]
Basolateral membrane	Secretion of conjugated bilirubin	Hepatocellular disease[c]
	Rate-limiting step	
Bile canaliculus	If distended, conjugated bilirubin leaks back	
Bile duct system	Concentrated in gallbladder	Obstructive jaundice[c]
Intestine	Converts bilirubin to many products	

[a]Conjugated bilirubin elevated, some increase in unconjugated.
[b]Unconjugated bilirubin elevated.
[c]Conjugated bilirubin elevated.

Table 12.3 Causes of jaundice

Hepatocellular disease	Conjugated bilirubin elevated
Obstructive jaundice	Conjugated bilirubin elevated
Jaundice of prematurity	Unconjugated bilirubin elevated
Gilbert's disease	Unconjugated bilirubin elevated (mild increase)
Haemolytic jaundice	Conjugated and unconjugated bilirubin elevated

K is given. The distension of the biliary system and bile canaliculi causes the enzyme serum alkaline phosphatase (SAP) to be released into the plasma, but the levels of other enzymes in plasma are normal or close to normal. There are no major abnormalities in the capacity of the liver for metabolism, storage, detoxification or synthesis (Table 12.4).

Hepatocellular diseases (for example, due to viral infection of the liver), by contrast, impair all liver functions. Viral hepatitis frequently starts with an initial low-grade fever and the first sign noticed may be dark urine. The conjugation of bilirubin may be reduced but conjugated bilirubin accumulates because the rate-limiting step is secretion into the bile canaliculus. Thus the capacity to conjugate is impaired but the bilirubin that accumulates is conjugated. Bilirubin does enter the bowel together with bile salts. There is little alteration in faecal colour or complex lipid absorption and there will be urobilinogen in the urine.

While all aspects of liver function are impaired, it depends on the severity as to which ones are manifest.

- Formation of blood coagulation proteins is reduced, leading to an increased INR that does not respond to an injection of vitamin K.
- Albumin synthesis is reduced but there is no immediate effect on plasma albumin because it has a large body pool and a prolonged half-life.
- Detoxification will be impaired and endogenous toxins and drugs handled by the liver will accumulate.
- The acute damage to the liver cells allows intracellular enzymes to enter the blood stream and so plasma liver enzymes are markedly elevated.
- Nitrogen metabolism will be impaired as the disease becomes more severe.

Carbohydrate metabolism and glycogen storage are only rarely impaired sufficiently to be clinically important. There

Table 12.4 Summary of major liver functions

Metabolic	Carbohydrate, protein, lipids
Detoxification	Endogenous and exogenous toxins; drugs
Synthesis	Proteins – albumin, blood coagulation products and gluconeogenesis
Storage	Glycogen, vitamin B_{12}
Bile formation	Bile salts, bilirubin, lipids

will also be abnormalities of lipid metabolism but these are not a problem acutely and are seen also in obstructive jaundice.

Besides the above types of jaundice, there are diseases that produce specific defects in the handling of bilirubin, such as Gilbert's disease, which causes mild bilirubin elevation of no serious consequence. Another defect occurs in premature infants. *In utero*, bilirubin produced in the fetus is cleared by the placenta. The enzyme glucuronyl-transferase does not develop until late in gestation. If an infant is premature, it lacks this enzyme and unconjugated bilirubin may accumulate. This is potentially serious as unconjugated bilirubin is lipid-soluble and can cross the blood–brain barrier, with toxic effects on the brain.

In chronic liver disease, the situation is markedly different to the situations described above. If there is no ongoing acute insult (for instance in a person with liver disease due to alcohol but now abstaining), the situation depends on the amount of liver tissue remaining and on the extent of disturbance of the hepatic architecture and circulation. The process that requires the greatest amount of liver tissue is albumin synthesis and a low plasma albumin may be the only biochemical defect seen. There is frequently no jaundice, although there is some elevation of bilirubin, and plasma liver enzymes are normal as there is no acute insult.

Oestrogen metabolism, as well as that of other steroid hormones such as aldosterone and glucocorticoids, may be impaired. The accumulation of oestrogen may cause spider naevi and, in males, feminization with female hair distribution, gynaecomastia and testicular atrophy. A major problem may result from the disturbance of the normal liver blood flow, which leads to an increase in portal venous pressure. Due to this increased portal venous pressure, anastomotic channels form connecting the portal system to the systemic circulation and bypassing the liver. The anastomotic circulation at the gastro-oesophageal region has thin-walled connections (oesophageal varices), which can bleed.

In a person with chronic liver disease there may be relatively few problems unless hepatic demand increases. If, however, plasma albumin falls below a critical level, which varies in different people, this precipitates a fall in circulating blood volume leading to low blood pressure and activation of the renin–angiotensin–aldosterone system. The resulting fluid retention is likely initially to be sequestrated in the abdominal cavity because of the elevated hydrostatic pressure at the venous ends of the capillaries in the portal system. As metabolism of aldosterone by the liver is also impaired, this intensifies the problem of fluid retention.

Problems of other types may also occur if the capacity of the liver is exceeded. Thus, an acute protein load may not be able to be readily handled and neurological problems may develop. Drug metabolism is often impaired and drug doses will need to be reduced. Toxins produced in the bowel may exceed the capacity of the liver to metabolize them or may bypass the liver by the anastomotic circulation and reach the brain. Bleeding from varices is a particular problem as it can lower blood pressure and reduce liver blood flow, as well as producing a large protein load due to digestion of haemoglobin in the bowel. If the person drinks alcohol or if there is a flare-up of hepatitis in a person with chronic liver disease, the signs, symptoms and biochemical changes of acute hepatocellular disease are superimposed on those of chronic liver disease.

KEY POINTS

- Key functions of the liver can be divided into metabolic, detoxification, synthetic, storage and bile formation.
- Bilirubin, the breakdown product of bile, is secreted by the liver calls into bile canaliculi.
- Bilirubin may be elevated due to excessive production, poor liver cell uptake, inadequate conjugation, inadequate secretion and blockage of the biliary system.
- The rate-limiting step in bilirubin metabolism is the secretion into the bile canaliculus.
- Absence of bile in the intestine leads to pale stools and failure of absorption of fat-soluble vitamins due to the absence of bile acids.
- Chronic liver disease may compensate for most functions and the major defect may be a low serum albumin.

ADDITIONAL READING

Braunwald E *et al.* (2001) *Harrison's Principles of Internal Medicine*, 15th edition. McGraw-Hill, New York.

Kelly DA (2002) Managing liver failure. *Postgraduate Medical Journal* **78**: 660–7.

Souhami RL & Moxham T (2002) *Textbook of Medicine*, 4th edition. Churchill Livingstone. London.

A series of 'funny turns'

CASE AND MCQS

Case introduction

A 65-year-old retired widow, Mrs G.K., who lives with her daughter, comes to seek advice late one morning. You saw her last 10 years ago, when she asked for a full check-up as a condition of employment in a secretarial agency. At that time, she was in good health and you have the details of that examination to compare with any present findings.

She says she has continued to enjoy good health until recently although over the last year she has become tired more easily, notices that she is often thirsty and has had occasional headaches that she describes as migraine. Several times re-cently she has had what she describes as 'funny turns'. Some of these have involved short periods of blurred vision ac-companied by numbness or tingling in one arm or her face; on another occasion she noticed that her arm felt both weak and numb.

These episodes have come on quickly and have lasted (she thinks) for only a few minutes. This morning, however, she had another occurrence shortly after she got out of bed and the symptoms have persisted, so now at 11.30 her sight is still blurred and her arm still feels numb.

Mrs K. is a moderately overweight (BMI 30), right-handed woman who is slightly flushed. She claims to drink occasion-ally and to have smoked moderately (10–12 cigarettes/day) since the age of 16.

Pulse rate is around 100 beats/min but varies consider-ably from beat to beat. Blood pressure by auscultation is 140/94 mmHg. Her jugular veins are not prominent and her heart sounds are normal.

She says that her right forearm and hand still feel numb although she is still able to detect and localize pinprick and light touch. She is rather clumsy at picking up a pin off your desk, but voluntary movements of her arm and fingers appear normal. Her elbow reflexes may be a little exaggerated.

You test Mrs K.'s visual fields using the simple technique of holding a piece of card over each of her eyes in turn and asking her to track a pen as you move it from left to right. The results are shown in Fig. 13.1.

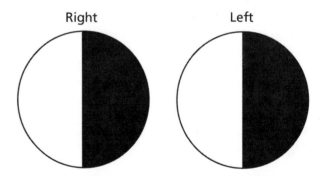

Fig. 13.1 Visual fields as recorded for Mrs K. The black areas represent loss of vision. There is total loss of vision in the medial half of the right and the lateral half of the patient's left visual field.

| Q1 | The pattern shown in Fig. 13.1 is consistent with a defect in: |

A. visual cortex
B. right optic tract
C. left optic tract
D. optic chiasma
E. left visual cortex

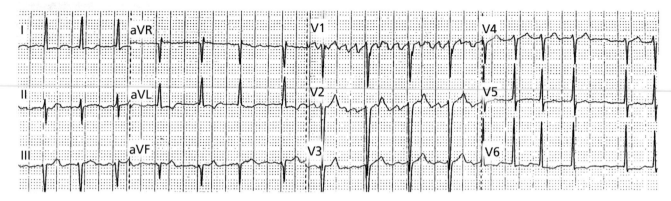

Fig. 13.2 12-lead ECG recorded from Mrs K. on first visit.

You record an ECG and the recording that you obtain is shown in Fig. 13.2 (above).

Q2 **This ECG record indicates:**

A. sinus arrhythmia
B. sinus tachycardia
C. atrial premature beats
D. atrial fibrillation
E. atrioventricular node failure

You take a blood sample for rough assessment of plasma glucose and lipid status using a digital strip reader. Mrs K. felt too ill to have any breakfast today, so you can regard these measurements as representing fasting levels.

The glucose readout indicates a plasma level of between 7 and 9 mmol/l (126–162 g/dl). The value you recorded 10 years previously was 6 mmol/l (108 mg/dl).

Q3 **The expected upper level for fasting plasma glucose in a normal individual is:**

A. 3 mmol/l (54 mg/dl)
B. 6 mmol/l (108 mg/dl)
C. 7 mmol/l (126 mg/dl)
D. 9 mmol/l (162 mg/dl)
E. 11 mmol/l (198 mg/dl)

Q4 **If there is elevated plasma glucose due to reduced cellular uptake, what will be the likely consequences?**

Mrs K.'s total blood cholesterol as measured using a strip reader is 6.8 mmol/l (263 mg/dl). This is higher than the recommended ceiling of 5.2 mmol/l (200 mg/dl) although it requires more accurate analysis of the different lipoprotein fractions in order for you to interpret it fully.

By the end of your consultation, Mrs. K.'s sight has cleared and the numbness in her arm is decreasing. The major concerns now are to identify the basis for her problem and decide on strategies to prevent a recurrence.

Let us look over the information that you have.

- Mrs K. now has elevated blood glucose, suggesting diabetes mellitus.
- Ten years ago, her glucose level was normal.
- Beta-cell failure is unlikely in a middle-aged or elderly person, so she may have non-insulin-dependent diabetes caused by insulin resistance.
- She also has elevated blood cholesterol (possibly as a response to the insulin resistance).
- She is an overweight smoker.

All the above factors increase her risk of atherosclerosis and thromboembolism. Before proceeding with her case, let us revise the functional roles of cholesterol in the body and how the formation of atheromatous plaques can lead to thromboembolism.

Q5 **Cholesterol is the precursor molecule for synthesis of all the following *except*:**

A. oestradiol
B. testosterone
C. cortisol
D. thyroxine
E. cholic acid

Q6 **Most of the cholesterol synthesized in the body is utilized for:**

A. formation of cell membranes
B. synthesis of bile salts
C. synthesis of gonadal hormones
D. synthesis of adrenocorticoid hormones
E. incorporation in the skin

Q7 The likelihood of atheroma formation is increased by:

A. high circulating LDL : HDL ratio
B. high circulating VLDL : HDL ratio
C. low circulating LDL : HDL ratio
D. low circulating VLDL : HDL ratio
E. none of the above

Q8 Regional blockage of vascular perfusion that occurs as a result of atherosclerosis is usually due to:

A. occlusion by local growth of an atheromatous plaque
B. occlusion by a dislodged atheromatous plaque
C. occlusion by a clot formed by blood contact with exposed collagen
D. inhibition of local vascular synthesis of nitric oxide
E. precipitation of calcium crystals in the vessel wall

Q9 The risk of atherosclerosis developing is decreased by:

A. hypothyroidism
B. iron overload
C. maleness
D. depletion of bile acids
E. all of the above

You also noted that Mrs K. has atrial fibrillation. This arrhythmia is known to increase the risk of thromboembolism independently of atherosclerosis.

Q10 Atrial fibrillation will increase the risk of intravascular thrombi because:

A. vibrations in the intra-atrial blood activate clotting factors
B. increased ejection turbulence causes platelet aggregation
C. reduced ejection turbulence prevents disruption of cell aggregates
D. reduced ventricular filling pressure prevents disruption of cell aggregates
E. reduced atrial ejection causes blood stasis in the atrial appendages

Mrs K.'s experiences of one arm becoming numb (*paraesthesia*) or weak (*hemiparesis*), together with the most recent occurrence of loss of half her visual fields (*hemianopsia*) are typical of brief local blockages in the cerebral circulation that are commonly known as transient ischaemic attacks (TIAs). By definition, these episodes last no longer than 24 hours. What she interpreted as migraine headaches might also have been the result of TIAs. These events are caused most com-

monly by thromboemboli, which in this case might have originated either from the atria or from the arterial tree.

Although the TIAs have apparently not left any persistent deficits, it is likely that at some time a longer lasting blockage will cause permanent brain damage (*stroke*). It is therefore important to reduce the risk factors as far as possible.

Mrs K.'s fasting glucose was only marginally outside the normal range. You order a glucose tolerance test in order to confirm her diabetes, together with a full plasma lipid analysis.

The glucose tolerance test assesses how efficiently glucose is removed into cells from the circulation. A dose of 1 g glucose per kg body mass is taken orally and the blood levels of both glucose and insulin are assessed at regular intervals over the ensuing several hours.

Q11 In a normal individual, blood glucose levels following oral administration of a glucose load will:

A. remain almost at resting values because of rapid cellular uptake
B. rise by around 30% and return to resting levels over around 2 hours
C. rise by around 30% and return to resting levels over around 3 hours
D. rise by around 100% and return to resting levels over around 2 hours
E. rise by around 100% and remain elevated for around 5 hours

The results confirm impaired cellular sensitivity to insulin with normal pancreatic capacity for insulin secretion. A variety of drugs are available which can be used to overcome insulin resistance but, as an initial approach, you decide to see whether weight loss will normalize insulin sensitivity without the need for drug therapy. You therefore book Mrs K. in for counselling with a dietician.

The results of her plasma lipid analysis are:

Total cholesterol	6.9 mmol/l
HDL	1.2 mmol/l
LDL	5.2 mmol/l
VLDL	0.5 mmol/l
Triglyceride	1.5 mmol/l

This shows a high LDL : HDL ratio of just over 5 and a total cholesterol well above the desirable 5.2 mmol/l (200 mg/dl). An ideal situation in an individual with no other risk factors for cardiovascular disease would involve an LDL value of less than 3.4 mmol/l (130 mg/dl) and an LDL : HDL ratio of 2–3. In somebody like Mrs K. who has a number of other factors predisposing her to atheroma, the target LDL would be even lower, with a ceiling of around 2.6 mmol/l (100 mg/dl).

On the basis of these data, you decide that it is important to reduce Mrs K.'s plasma cholesterol as a matter of urgency.

In theory, diet and weight loss can be used to achieve this in many patients but, since she is already at high risk of cerebrovascular damage, you decide to use pharmacological treatment with a statin.

The statins are drugs that reduce hepatic cholesterol synthesis by inhibiting 3-hydroxyl-3-methylglutaryl (HMG) CoA reductase – the enzyme responsible for normal feedback control of cholesterol production in response to changes in plasma cholesterol concentration. In fact, the therapeutic effect of statins is preferentially to reduce circulating LDL cholesterol rather than total cholesterol. This is because reduced cholesterol synthesis leads to compensatory induction of hepatocyte LDL receptors.

You also wish to lower the likelihood of further thrombus formation, particularly in view of her atrial fibrillation. The most commonly used drugs for this purpose are the coumarin-type anticoagulants and aspirin.

Q12 The coumarin drugs have antithrombotic activity because they:

A. activate plasminogen
B. prevent formation of prothrombin
C. inhibit platelet aggregation
D. prevent activation of factor XII
E. prevent formation of thromboplastin

Q13 Aspirin has antithrombotic activity because it:

A. dilutes the blood by causing water retention
B. dilates blood vessels by inhibiting prostaglandin synthesis
C. dilates blood vessels by inhibiting oxidative phosphorylation
D. prevents platelet aggregation by inhibiting thromboxane synthesis
E. prevents thrombin formation by inhibiting prothrombin activation

Warfarin is the usual drug of choice for patients with uncomplicated atrial fibrillation because it is a more powerful anticlotting agent than aspirin. In this case, however, Mrs K.'s atheroma and history of TIAs means that her blood vessels are more susceptible to damage than normal. She is therefore at risk of haemorrhages if the capacity of her blood to clot is depressed dramatically. For this reason, you prescribe her aspirin (100 mg/day) along with the statin and advise her to stop smoking immediately. Any decisions on whether to treat her insulin resistance and mild hypertension with drugs will be held over until you see whether diet alone has any effect.

One week later, you receive a call from Mrs. K.'s daughter. Her mother collapsed when getting breakfast and has been taken to the local hospital.

When you arrive, you find Mrs K. is conscious and alert, with no headache or signs of confusion.

- She understands what people say to her and can speak in full sentences, but she is unable to enunciate words clearly (*dysarthria*).
- She has no visual disturbance and her pupils are even and respond normally to light.
- She is able to wrinkle her forehead and close her eyes, but cannot open her mouth wide. When she is asked to stick her tongue out, it curves to the right; when she is asked to smile, she can move only the left side of her mouth.
- She can raise her right upper arm to the level of her shoulder but no higher. Her right forearm is almost completely paralysed and she cannot move the fingers of that hand. However, cutaneous sensation on arm and hand seem normal
- She can flex both legs but is not able to wriggle her right foot or flex the toes on that side as strongly as on the left side, and her right leg cannot support her when standing.

Q14 The distribution of deficits indicates that the site of damage is:

A. cerebellum
B. midbrain
C. supplementary motor cortex
D. primary motor cortex
E. thalamus

Q15 This site of damage suggests that the main artery involved is:

A. frontal branch of anterior cerebral artery
B. frontoparietal branch of anterior cerebral artery
C. parietal branch of middle cerebral artery
D. parietal branch of posterior cerebral artery
E. temporal branch of posterior cerebral artery

Q16 Note that although there is damage to the motor outflows to face and both upper and lower limbs, there is a very uneven distribution in the severity of effects, with more impairment of finger movement than limb movement. Why is this pattern seen?

CT scanning (Fig. 13.3) confirms the site of the infarct as being in the central territory of the anterior cerebral artery, and also reveals several small, old infarcts. There is no evidence of haemorrhage contributing to the present brain ischaemia.

Magnetic resonance angiography shows some narrowing of the bifurcations of the internal carotid artery with

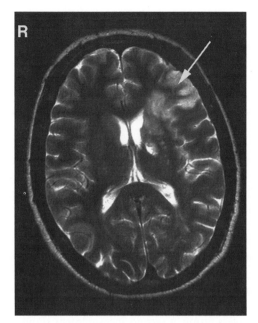

Fig. 13.3 CT scan from Mrs K. The infarcted area of brain is arrowed.

anterior and middle cerebral arteries, probably indicating atheroma.

You prescribe streptokinase so as to help break down the occluding thrombus.

Q17 | Streptokinase acts as a thrombolytic agent because it:

A. changes the conformation of plasminogen
B. converts plasminogen to plasmin
C. digests fibrin
D. inactivates thrombin
E. sequesters calcium ions

Q18 | The activation of plasminogen that occurs during normal thrombolysis originates from:

A. plasminogen activator released by endothelial cells
B. plasminogen activator released by megakaryocytes
C. plasminogen activator synthesized within the fibrin clot
D. degradation of plasminogen inhibitor by circulating enzymes
E. conjugation with antithrombin

Once a stroke has occurred, minimizing the risk factors becomes an even greater concern. Since hypertension is a known risk factor for stroke, one aspect of care has to be pharmacological reduction of blood pressure to normal levels.

With Mrs K. and all cases of severe stroke, it is important not to lower blood pressure too rapidly. In regions of the brain that are ischaemic, the arterioles no longer respond to altered input pressure with autoregulatory adjustments of resistance, so a sudden fall of blood pressure may cause a drastic fall in cerebral perfusion and further ischaemic damage.

Q19 | In a normal person, autoregulation maintains cerebral blood flow virtually constant over a range of mean arterial input pressures of about:

A. 0–100 mmHg
B. 50–100 mmHg
C. 50–150 mmHg
D. 100–150 mmHg
E. 50–200 mmHg

Q20 | Autoregulation in the cerebral circulation is controlled primarily by the local concentration of:

A. nitric oxide
B. protons
C. inorganic phosphate
D. adenine breakdown products
E. oxygen

Lowering blood pressure by any means probably lowers the risk of another stroke but some studies suggest that drugs with certain mechanisms of action may confer a greater benefit than others, perhaps because they have additional actions. One class of antihypertensive that has been suggested to be especially effective in protecting against stroke is the calcium-channel blocking agents such as verapamil and nifedipine. These agents act primarily by inactivating voltage-operated calcium channels.

Q21 | Inactivation of voltage-operated calcium channels reduces blood pressure because it reduces:

A. action potential-mediated calcium entry into cardiac muscle
B. calcium liberation from cardiac sarcoplasmic reticulum
C. calcium liberation from vascular smooth muscle sarcoplasmic reticulum
D. noradrenaline-mediated calcium entry into vascular smooth muscle
E. action potential-mediated calcium entry into vascular smooth muscle

By the third day post admission, Mrs K. can move her right hand slightly but still cannot produce lower facial movements. After a further 3 days, she can stand and walk a few steps. By two weeks post admission, she is able to move her hand normally and grip objects well and she can walk around the room without support. There is still facial and limb muscle weakness but this is not as pronounced as previously; her smile is symmetrical and tongue movement is normal.

She is discharged into her daughter's care and enrolled in a rehabilitation programme. This helps her to cope with her reduced motor function but she has no further return of motor capacity over the next year.

MCQ ANSWERS AND FEEDBACK

1.B. Information from the lateral half of the ipsilateral retina and the medial half of the contralateral retina travels in the optic tract to the lateral geniculate and from there to visual cortex via the optic irradiation. Damage to tract, geniculate or irradiation would produce the pattern illustrated. However, because of the spread of projections across the visual cortex, a lesion at the cortical level would not produce clear interference with one half of the visual field. Figure 13.4 shows a diagram of the visual system to remind you of the circuitry.

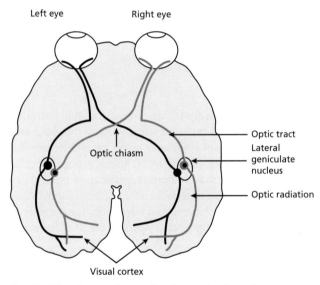

Fig. 13.4 The visual pathway, showing projections of information from each half of each retinal field to the visual cortex.

2.D. Absence of clear atrial P waves suggests absence of an atrial pacemaker, but P waves are sometimes not well delineated in all leads even in a normal heart. What definitively indicates atrial fibrillation is a combination of no P waves with a relatively high and quite irregular frequency of ventricular excitation. During atrial fibrillation, action potentials arrive at the atrioventricular node at quite irregular intervals because they are travelling along a variety of pathways within the atrial muscle. Atrial premature beats (extrasystoles) are due to occasional additional action potentials being generated from an intra-atrial ectopic focus, so they would be seen as irregular extra beats superimposed on a regular underlying rhythm. The present record shows no evidence of such basic regularity. Atrial fibrillation is the most common arrhythmia, with an incidence of around 1 in 200 in the general population and 1 in 20 in those more than 65 years old.

3.B. In most people, fasting plasma glucose is around 5–5.5 mmol/l. Current World Health Organization guidelines specify that a value higher than 7 mmol/l is diagnostic of diabetes in individuals who have symptoms of this disorder and highly suggestive in individuals without symptoms. In the symptomless group, a second measurement should be carried out on another day. In cases where fasting glucose levels are only just above the upper limit of normal, a glucose tolerance test may also be carried out, to confirm whether cellular glucose uptake is disturbed.

4. Increased plasma glucose has several deleterious consequences. As the proximal tubules have a transport maximum for glucose reabsorption of around 21 mmol/min (375 mg/min), plasma glucose concentrations above 17 mmol/l (300 mg/dl) at a normal glomerular filtration rate (GFR) of 125 ml/min will result in glucose being retained in the tubular fluid and lead to osmotic diuresis, with loss from the body of water, electrolytes and glucose itself. The presence of glucose in the urine encourages the growth of microorganisms, leading to urinary tract infections. Excess glucose in the extracellular environment will directly increase extracellular osmolality, leading to loss of water from cells and disruption of intracellular machinery. A deficiency in cellular availability of glucose for energy production will result in mobilization of lipids and elevation of plasma cholesterol. As chronically high blood lipids predispose to atherosclerosis, diabetic patients are at increased risk of myocardial infarcts, peripheral vascular disease and stroke.

5.D. Cholesterol is the precursor molecule for all steroid hormones and for bile salts. Thyroxine is a catechol molecule, resembling adrenaline and noradrenaline (epinephrine and norepinephrine) in structure.

6.B. Cholesterol is essential for many purposes in the body. It is the precursor for all steroid hormones, it constitutes the essential water-resistant layer in the skin that prevents dehydration and, together with phospholipids, it makes up the lipid layer of all cell membranes. While each of these roles is vital to survival, the total amount of newly synthesized cholesterol that they require is small. Around 80% of all cholesterol synthesized by the liver is used to form the cholic acid precursor of bile salts.

7.A. Most of the circulating cholesterol is carried in either high-density lipoproteins (HDL) or low-density lipoproteins (LDL). The role of LDL is to deliver cholesterol to cells; the role of HDL is to transport cholesterol to the liver for bile salt production. So a high LDL : HDL ratio represents a situation where there is likely to be net tissue deposition of cholesterol while a low LDL : HDL ratio is indicative of net clearance of tissue cholesterol. The very low-density lipoproteins (VLDL) carry mainly triglyceride and only a small amount of cholesterol. Although there is a weak correlation between high VLDL and cardiovascular risk, this is probably because high VLDL levels are usually associated with lower circulating levels of HDL.

8.C. Atheromatous plaques form when local accumulation of LDL causes local inflammation in the subendothelial layer of an artery. This stimulates the laying down of new smooth muscle and fibrous connective tissue (*sclera*) below the endothelium, endothelial damage with reduced nitric oxide production and later infiltration of the site by calcium crystals. Collectively, these events narrow the arterial lumen and reduce arterial wall distensibility. On occasions, the endothelial damage is so severe that the surface of the plaque itself becomes exposed to the bloodstream.

Contact of blood with the connective tissue activates factor XII and platelet aggregation, resulting in an intravascular clot (*thrombus*). The clot may continue to grow in size until it blocks the vessel at its site of formation, or it may become dislodged to form an embolus and block a smaller vessel downstream. The plaque itself is firmly embedded in the vessel wall and could not be dislodged, although sometimes a plaque can encroach on the vessel lumen so much that it obstructs blood flow past that site.

9.D. If the normal recycling of bile salts via the enterohepatic circulation is prevented, production of new bile salts has to increase. This involves hepatic conversion of cholesterol to bile salts and a compensatory increase in hepatic LDL receptors, to provide hepatic uptake of LDL as a source of additional cholesterol. The end result is therefore a fall in plasma LDL. Ingestion of anion-exchange resins that sequester bile salts in the intestinal lumen is a highly effective treatment for patients who have severe hypercholesterolaemia, although the side-effects on digestive function limit the general use of these agents for reducing plasma LDL.

A variety of factors predispose to atherosclerosis even in the presence of normal plasma LDL, HDL and cholesterol. In ad-

dition to the associations with smoking, obesity and diabetes that have been mentioned earlier, high blood levels of iron, low thyroid hormone levels and an absence of female gonadal hormones are all associated with more plaque formation. The effect of iron is probably due to pro-inflammatory effects of free radicals liberated by oxidation of ferrous to ferric state. Low thyroid hormone increases plasma cholesterol, probably because of effects on enzymic processing of lipids. It is uncertain whether the higher incidence of atherogenesis in men and post-menopausal women is due to a pro-atherogenic effect of androgens or to an anti-atherogenic effect of oestrogens.

10.E. The absence of atrial contraction is associated with some blood being trapped in the atrial appendages rather than being continually mixed and recycled. Since clots and cell aggregates are more likely to form in stationary blood, the presence of atrial fibrillation greatly increases the risk of thromboembolism. About 10% of strokes are secondary to these intracardiac emboli.

11.B. Typically, oral ingestion of 1 g/kg glucose elevates plasma glucose from around 5 mmol/l (90 mg/dl) to around 7 mmol/l (130 mg/dl) within 45–60 minutes and the level returns to its resting value over the next hour. In fact, there is normally a fall to slightly below the fasting value because of the relatively long half-life of insulin in the circulation. In diabetics, plasma glucose rises by up to 100%, the level remains high for several hours and there is no recovery overshoot. Simultaneous measurements of insulin levels allow discrimination between type I (no insulin rise) and type II (normal or exaggerated insulin rise) diabetes.

12.B. Warfarin and similar coumarin drugs bind to vitamin K in the liver and prevent formation of several clotting factors – prothrombin and factors VII, IX and X. All of these factors depend on binding of calcium ions for conversion to their active state and vitamin K is essential for formation of the calcium-binding site.

13.D. Platelet aggregation depends on secretion of ADP and thromboxane A_2. As thromboxane formation is catalysed by cyclo-oxygenase, the potent inhibitory effect of aspirin on this enzyme reduces the efficiency of aggregation considerably. Aspirin can cause water retention and vascular relaxation, but only at high doses of several grams per day such as are used to treat inflammatory responses in patients with rheumatoid conditions. The dose required to reduce platelet aggregation (300 mg or less) is even lower than that usually taken for headache (around 600 mg). In patients who have suffered previous strokes, some trials indicate that regular low-dose aspirin reduces the risk of further events by at least 50% and that no additional benefit is seen when aspirin is supplemented by anticoagulants like warfarin. However, in patients who do not have clear risk factors or have suffered previous TIAs, it is debatable whether the antithrombotic benefits of aspirin outweigh the increased risk of haemorrhage.

14.D. The presentation is characteristic of damage to the primary motor cortex. Lesions in supplementary motor cortex or cerebellum would cause loss of motor control but not motor paralysis. Lesions in thalamus or midbrain would be likely to affect visual and somatosensory systems as well as motor outflow.

15.B. The frontoparietal branch of anterior and the frontal branch of middle cerebral artery provide blood supply to the primary motor cortex, while the parietal branch of middle cerebral artery supplies the somatosensory cortex. The territory of the posterior cerebral artery is nowhere near motor cortex. Figure 13.5 shows the regional distributions of each division of the cerebral arterial tree (but remember that there is some crossover of territories along the margins of these divisions).

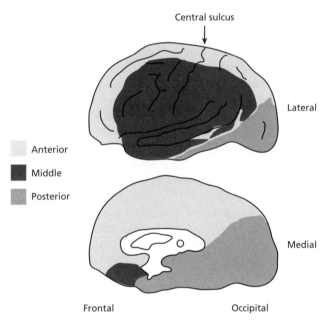

Fig. 13.5 Territories of blood supply to the brain from anterior, middle and posterior cerebral arteries. The more caudal regions of the brain are not shown as they are supplied by the vertebral arteries.

16. The parts of the body that are most affected by ischaemia of either motor or sensory cortices are those which have the largest somatotopic cortical projections. Thus, only the most severe degrees of cortical ischaemia affect sensorimotor function in the trunk, while far less disruption is needed to impair movement and sensation in fingers, toes and mouth.

17.A. Streptokinase is a protein derived from beta-haemolytic streptococci. It has no inherent enzymic activity, but forms a stable complex with plasminogen that alters the conformation of that molecule so as to expose the active site. This allows cleavage of the plasminogen to form free plasmin. Plasmin digests the fibrin clot and also inactivates some clotting factors, reducing further coagulation. High doses of streptokinase are needed for a therapeutic effect because plasma always contains antibodies against streptococcal proteins, resulting from previous infections,

18.A. Thrombin and other substances produced during the clotting process stimulate release of plasminogen activator from the adjacent endothelium. This process occurs only slowly, so clots are not usually broken down until 1–2 days after their formation. However, it is essential that this process occurs continually. Tiny clots that obstruct skin microcirculatory vessels are being formed all the time by local physical trauma; the continual dissolution of these is necessary in order to prevent progressive loss of skin perfusion and impairment of temperature regulation.

19.C. The lower limit of input pressure at which autoregulatory adjustments occur is 50–60 mmHg. Pressure gradients lower than this are not sufficient to maintain perfusion even when the arterioles are maximally dilated, In normotensive individuals, the highest input pressure that can be compensated for by autoregulatory mechanisms is 140–150 mmHg. However, in individuals with chronic hypertension, structural changes in the arterial wall can result in autoregulation at pressures up to 200 mmHg.

20.B. Large changes in interstitial or intravascular concentrations of any of these substances will relax arteriolar smooth muscle but, in the cerebral circulation, only interstitial proton levels vary enough under physiological circumstances to be able to act as an autoregulatory factor. The protons originate as CO_2 produced from neuronal metabolism but this is rapidly broken down under the influence of interstitial carbonic anhydrase. Vascular autoregulation relies on the fact that all cellular metabolites are vasodilator, with their interstitial concentration and dilator effect being inversely related to the rate at which they are washed away into the bloodstream. In the case of the cerebral circulation, this situation can be mimicked by altering arterial P_{CO_2}. In consequence, if one causes hypocapnia by hyperventilating then cerebral vasoconstriction occurs and oxygen delivery to the brain may fall sufficiently to produce a feeling of dizziness.

21.E. Smooth muscle cells contain very little sarcoplasmic reticulum and so virtually all the calcium needed for sarcomere activation during contraction must be obtained by diffusion down its concentration gradient from the extracellular fluid. The channels required for this are the same channels as carry the inward current during the depolarizing phase of the muscle action potential.

CASE REVIEW

What we term as stroke is defined as focal damage to an area of the brain caused by an acute fall in blood supply. The clinical presentation characteristically involves muscle weakness on one side of the body, often with inability to speak clearly. Brief cerebrovascular deficits that cause symptoms lasting for less than 24 hours are arbitrarily termed transient ischaemic attacks (TIAs) rather than strokes. However, the causes are identical and TIAs often precede longer lasting attacks, so it is more realistic to classify them as mini-strokes rather than as a separate category.

Stroke is the third most common cause of death in developed countries, after cancer and myocardial infarction. Each year, over 300 000 strokes occur in the USA and 140 000 occur in the UK, with around 30% of these patients dying as a result and a high percentage of the survivors having some degree of permanent disability.

Most strokes (85%) are due to regional interference with arterial blood flow by a local thrombus that develops on an exposed atheromatous plaque (*stenosis*) or by blockage with a blood-borne thrombus (*embolism*). Stenosis is most likely just downstream of an arterial bifurcation, probably because the branching produces flow characteristics that predispose to endothelial damage. Emboli originate most commonly from dislodged atheromatous thrombi. About a quarter of cases, however, involve thrombi that form within the heart chambers because inefficient contraction results in blood pooling; typically in patients who have long-standing atrial fibrillation or cardiac failure.

Since the probability of an obstructive blockage will be related to the volume of blood that is delivered to the vessel, the majority of ischaemic strokes affect the territory of the artery that carries the highest proportion of cerebral perfusion, the middle cerebral artery. For this reason, unilateral impairment of motor function is a typical result.

Most of the 15% of strokes that are not due to obstruction are caused by rupture of a small cerebral artery. Intracerebral haemorrhage not only produces local neuronal damage but also obstructs blood flow to more remote areas because of the increased extravascular pressure. Administration of anti-haemostatic agents like aspirin or anticoagulants might be valuable in a patient with thrombosis but fatal in a patient with intracranial bleeding. Distinguishing between the two causes by brain imaging is therefore a mandatory part of patient management, with computed tomographic (CT) scanning being the technique of choice for early assessment under most circumstances.

The incidence of stroke is highly age-dependent. They are rare below the age of 40 years and progressively more common over the age range 50–80 years. Hypertension greatly increases the risk of stroke, probably mainly because of shear stress-induced endothelial damage resulting in atheroma. Not surprisingly, therefore, a number of other factors that are known to increase the likelihood of hypertension and of arteriosclerosis also increase the risk of stroke – for example smoking, diabetes mellitus, obesity and elevated plasma LDL cholesterol.

Satisfactory treatment of the stroke patient must take into consideration a wide range of issues and involves a wide range of resources and skills. At present, effective pharmacotherapy is restricted mainly to addressing the circulatory defects. In the future, however, it should become possible to target directly the processes that cause neuronal damage itself, using drugs that reduce free radical accumulation or modulate intraneuronal signalling pathways. Depending on the area of brain affected, there may be impairment of neural control of a variety of endocrine and autonomic functions. Peripheral effects of impaired motor function can also contribute substantially to post-stroke morbidity, as loss of coordinated swallowing can lead to aspiration pneumonia and immobility predisposes to venous thromboembolism. Finally, optimizing the process of rehabilitation involves complex multidisciplinary care.

KEY POINTS

- Brain damage caused by local reduction of cerebral blood flow (stroke) is a common event in older populations and represents the third most frequent cause of death in Western countries.
- The majority of strokes are due to arterial blockage by a thrombus originating in the heart or on an exposed atheromatous plaque.
- The most common territory affected is that supplied by the middle cerebral artery, with unilateral motor impairment being the characteristic result.
- Treatment of the stroke patient is a complex process that involves managing the acute central and peripheral deficits, reducing the risk of recurrent events and a multidisciplinary approach to rehabilitation.

ADDITIONAL READING

Barnett HJM, Bogousslavsky J & Meldrum H (2003) *Ischemic Stroke* (*Advances in Neurology* volume 92). Lippincott Williams & Wilkins, Philadelphia.

Bath PMW & Lees KR (2000) ABC of arterial and venous disease: acute stroke. *British Medical Journal* **320**: 920–3.

Brown LC, Johnson JA, Majumdar SR, Tsuyuki RT & McAlister FA (2004) Evidence of suboptimal management of cardiovascular risk in patients with type 2 diabetes mellitus and symptomatic atherosclerosis. *Canadian Medical Association Journal* **171**: 1189–92.

Pedelty L & Gorelick PB (2004) Chronic management of blood pressure after stroke. *Hypertension* **44**: 1–5.

Viles-Gonzalez JF, Anand SX, Valdiviezo C *et al.* (2004) Update in athero-thrombotic disease. *Mount Sinai Journal of Medicine* **71**: 197–208.

Four weeks at high altitude

CASE AND MCQS

Case introduction

Kathy B., a final-year medical student from Dublin, is organizing a six-week visit to the Andes for the Irish Medical Students' Association. During this trip, the participants plan to stay at a high-altitude research station, where they can monitor their physiological responses to high altitude and undertake comparative measurements on long-term inhabitants at the same altitudes.

The expedition will consist of a maximum of 10 students, together with a staff member who is a specialist in travel medicine. There are initially 14 applicants, all in the final 2 years of medical studies in Ireland (age range 23–34 years, mean 26) and coming from a variety of ethnic backgrounds.

Preparations for the trip include screening all applicants to make sure that nobody has any underlying medical condition that will be a problem at high altitude. A full blood screen is carried out, together with specific tests that identify some relatively common abnormalities of haemoglobin structure.

The routine blood screen is performed in a Coulter counter, which provides automated analysis of several parameters. Some of these are listed below together with typical normal values for young healthy adults:

Red cell count	men 4.5–6.0×10^9/ml; women 3.5–5.4×10^9/ml
Haemoglobin	men 13.0–17.0 g/dl; women 12.0–16.0 g/dl
Haematocrit	men 40–50%; women 35–49%
Mean cell volume	82–95 fl
Mean cell haemoglobin	27–32 pg
Reticulocytes	0.2–2.0%

Q1 Women characteristically have lower haematocrits than men because:

A. oestrogens stimulate formation of plasma albumin
B. testosterone upregulates erythropoiesis
C. women have regular menstrual blood loss
D. women have less capacity to store iron
E. erythrocyte lifespan is shorter in women

Two students are identified as having abnormal blood profiles that may interfere with their suitability for inclusion on the trip. One of these is Julie G., whose family comes from Naples. Her results are as follows:

Red cell count	5.8×10^9/ml
Haemoglobin	11.0 g/dl
Mean cell volume	70 fl
Mean cell haemoglobin	19 pg
Reticulocytes	6%

Q2 The diagnosis is:

A. hypochromic, normocytic anaemia
B. hypochromic, macrocytic anaemia
C. hypochromic, microcytic anaemia
D. normochromic, microcytic anaemia
E. normochromic, normocytic anaemia

Q3 This classification is compatible with:

A. beta-thalassaemia
B. iron deficiency
C. pernicious anaemia
D. any of the above
E. either A or B only

Julie's blood is tested further, using electrophoresis to characterize the globin chains. This confirms that she has a mild form of *beta-thalassaemia* (beta-thalassaemia minor). Carrier status of beta-thalassaemias is common in a belt across the Mediterranean and northern Africa through the Middle East and India, to Southeast Asia, with gene frequencies of up to 20% in some parts of Italy and Greece. Julie's disease is heterozygous and does not cause severe enough anaemia to be dangerous, but the homozygous disease is a substantial health care problem in the endemic areas.

The second student with an unusual blood profile is Carl B., a student from London. Carl has normal red cell numbers and haemoglobin concentration but haemoglobin testing with a precipitation assay reveals that he is heterozygous for the sickle cell gene. The gene is extremely common in people of West African descent, with an incidence of around 10–20% in black USA and UK populations. It results in a single amino acid substitution in the beta-globin chain, causing polymerization of the haemoglobin molecule when it is deoxygenated and especially when the environment is hyperosmotic. As a result, the erythrocytes become physically distorted, with conversion of the normal biconcave cell profile into a stiff elongated shape.

 Q4 **You would predict that this structural alteration of the erythrocyte would be associated with:**

A. increased red cell turnover
B. reduced blood viscosity
C. increased peripheral perfusion
D. reduced reticulocyte counts
E. none of the above

Q5 **In view of the consequences of sickling, it would be dangerous for Carl to be exposed to a hypoxic environment. Is the main danger related to his capacity for oxygen carriage, or to other factors?**

Q6 **Sickling is most likely in an environment that is hyperosmotic as well as hypoxic. In view of this, which of the following do you think is most likely to be produced by hypoxia in an individual with sickle cell trait?**

A. bone pain
B. coronary infarction
C. stroke
D. polyuria
E. respiratory oedema

Carl is advised that he cannot join the trip and he is counselled about the circumstances under which adverse effects might be precipitated by hypoxia. In addition to general anaesthesia, these include periods at even relatively moderate altitudes around 2000–2500 m (6500–8200 ft) and dehydration. Long-haul air travel is therefore potentially dangerous for somebody with sickle cell trait.

Julie's slight anaemia is not sufficient to reduce her oxygen carriage substantially and she could probably take part in the trip without difficulty, but she decides against it.

The final party consists of nine students and the medical officer. One of these students reports that she has asthma and sometimes suffers an acute attack during exercise on cold days. She is concerned that the cold, dry conditions in the Andes might be a problem.

Q7 **Acute asthma during exercise is triggered by:**

A. systemic hypoxia due to increased oxygen consumption
B. dehydration of airway mucosa due to increased air flow
C. stimulation of airway chemoreceptors by increased inhalation of allergens
D. direct bronchoconstrictor effect of increased oxygen tension
E. airway shrinkage due to reduced circulating plasma volume

In theory, the fact that exercise can precipitate an asthmatic attack suggests that asthma-prone individuals should avoid high altitude. In reality, they seem less likely to respond poorly at altitude than at sea level. It is possible that the asthmogenic effect of dry air is more than compensated for by the presence of fewer allergens and pollutants at high altitude.

All members of the group take their baseline haematological and cardiorespiratory data with them, together with some portable equipment for field measurement of respiratory and haematological function. In Kathy's case, the baseline information she has includes:

Haematocrit	41%
Haemoglobin	12.2 g/dl
Arterial $P\text{CO}_2$	40 mmHg (5.4 kPa)
Arterial $P\text{O}_2$	96 mmHg (12.8 kPa)
Arterial pH	7.41
Arterial bicarbonate	26 mmol/l
Functional residual capacity	2.2 litres
Resting minute ventilation	5.8 litres

The party flies from London to Lima (altitude sea level) and transfers to La Oroya research station by light plane. La Oroya is 3700 m (11 500 ft) above sea level, a similar altitude to many resorts in the Rocky Mountains and in the European Alps (Fig. 14.1). The students arrive at 09.15 hours.

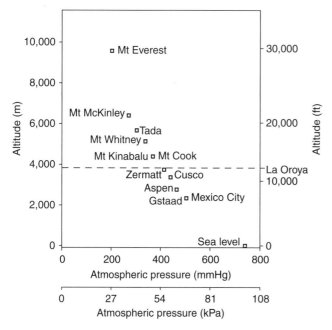

Fig. 14.1 Altitudes above sea level of some well-known locations. The destination for Kathy's trip is shown by the dashed line.

Q8 The barometric pressure at 3700 m (11 500 ft) altitude is 480 mmHg (64 kPa). What is the atmospheric P_{O_2}?

A. 480 mmHg (64 kPa)
B. 433 mmHg (58 kPa)
C. 380 mmHg (51 kPa)
D. 100 mmHg (13 kPa)
E. 53 mmHg (7 kPa)

Q9 With this atmospheric P_{O_2}, what would Kathy's P_{AO_2} be if she continued to ventilate at the same minute volume as at sea level?

A. 100 mmHg (13 kPa)
B. 90 mmHg (12 kPa)
C. 50 mmHg (6.5 kPa)
D. 20 mmHg (2.7 kPa)
E. cannot be calculated without further data

Immediately Kathy gets out of the plane she notices that she is breathing heavily and that by the time she has walked to the arrival hall she feels out of breath. The rest of the group have similar responses. As soon as they have been able to unpack their equipment, they make respiratory and blood gas measurements. The time is now 10.15 hours.

Kathy's measured minute ventilation at this time is 9 l/min.

Q10 This immediate elevation of minute ventilation at altitude, relative to the pattern at sea level, is due to:

A. stimulation of peripheral chemoreceptors by hypoxia
B. stimulation of central chemoreceptors by hypoxia
C. stimulation of peripheral chemoreceptors by hypocapnia
D. elevated metabolic rate due to the low ambient temperature
E. none of the above

Q11 If an arterial blood sample from Kathy was taken at this time, which of the following sets of data would you expect?

A. P_{O_2} 110 mmHg (14.7 kPa), P_{CO_2} 40 mmHg (5.4 kPa), pH 7.40
B. P_{O_2} 110 mmHg (14.7 kPa), P_{CO_2} 35 mmHg (4.7 kPa), pH 7.55
C. P_{O_2} 70 mmHg (9.3 kPa), P_{CO_2} 35 mmHg (4.7 kPa), pH 7.40
D. P_{O_2} 56 mmHg (7.5 kPa), P_{CO_2} 40 mmHg (5.4 kPa), pH 7.40
E. P_{O_2} 56 mmHg (7.5 kPa), P_{CO_2} 35 mmHg (4.7 kPa), pH 7.55

By 3 hours after arrival, Kathy has toured the research unit and met the staff. It is lunchtime, but several members of the group, including Kathy, have begun to feel ill. She has a headache, nausea and vomiting and recognizes that she probably has developed a syndrome called 'acute mountain sickness'. All members of the group were advised to dose themselves with a carbonic anhydrase inhibitor (acetazolamide) for several days before travelling to minimize the symptoms of this syndrome. Kathy forgot to take her pills.

Q12 Carbonic anhydrase is involved in:

A. exocrine pancreatic secretion
B. renal tubular recycling of filtered bicarbonate
C. erythrocytic carriage of CO_2
D. all of the above
E. none of the above

Q13 If inhibition of carbonic anhydrase lessens the symptoms of acute mountain sickness, this suggests that the symptoms are caused by:

A. metabolic alkalosis due to renal bicarbonate retention
B. respiratory alkalosis due to hypocapnia
C. metabolic acidosis due to renal bicarbonate loss
D. dehydration due to increased ventilation
E. hypoxia

Kathy stays in bed until the next morning and finds that her headache and nausea have almost gone. When she gets up, she also notices that she does not become as breathless when moving around as occurred yesterday, although it is still an effort to climb stairs.

She finds that her minute ventilation is now 12 l/min. She takes a finger prick blood sample and finds that her haematocrit has risen from its normal value of 41% to 45%.

<table>
<tr><td>**Q14**</td><td>**The overnight changes in breathlessness, ventilatory volume and symptoms are due to:**</td></tr>
</table>

A. sensitization of central chemoreceptor drive by local bicarbonate diffusion
B. sensitization of central chemoreceptor drive by CO_2 retention
C. restoration of systemic acid–base balance by renal compensation
D. increased peripheral chemoreceptor stimulation by persistent hypoxia
E. increased peripheral chemoreceptor stimulation due to ventilation/perfusion mismatching

<table>
<tr><td>**Q15**</td><td>**The rise in haematocrit since leaving sea level can be explained by:**</td></tr>
</table>

A. hypocapnia causing peripheral vasodilation
B. renal hypoxia stimulating erythropoietin secretion
C. increased ventilation leading to respiratory water loss
D. reduced atmospheric pressure causing peripheral venous pooling
E. none of the above

<table>
<tr><td>**Q16**</td><td>**If Kathy had another arterial sample analysed at this time, which set of data would you expect?**</td></tr>
</table>

A. Po_2 64 mmHg (8.5 kPa), Pco_2 25 mmHg (3.3 kPa), pH 7.40
B. Po_2 64 mmHg (8.5 kPa), Pco_2 30 mmHg (4.0 kPa), pH 7.55
C. Po_2 64 mmHg (8.5 kPa), Pco_2 35 mmHg (4.7 kPa), pH 7.40
D. Po_2 56 mmHg (7.5 kPa), Pco_2 35 mmHg (4.7 kPa), pH 7.40
E. Po_2 56 mmHg (7.5 kPa), Pco_2 25 mmHg (3.3 kPa), pH 7.55

Over the next few days, Kathy becomes progressively less breathless on exertion, while her minute ventilation remains constant at 12 l/min.

<table>
<tr><td>**Q17**</td><td>**This improved adaptation is due primarily to:**</td></tr>
</table>

A. increased synthesis of red blood cells
B. increased erythrocyte content of 2,3 diphosphoglycerate (DPG)
C. increased erythrocyte content of haemoglobin
D. all of the above
E. both A and B

The research activities in which Kathy is involved show that the staff who have been living on this station for about 12 months have blood gas values similar to hers, but have haematocrits of 55–60%. She also notices that their ECG patterns are quite unlike anything she has seen before, even in the cardiology clinic. In particular, QRS waveforms in the thoracic leads V_1–V_6 look very unusual (Fig. 14.2).

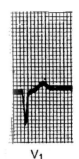 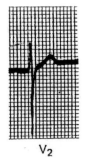 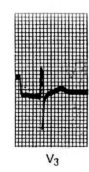 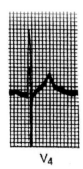 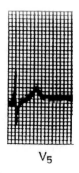 

| V_1 | V_2 | V_3 | V_4 | V_5 | V_6 |

Fig. 14.2 Thoracic lead ECG records obtained from one of the La Oroya research staff (J.X.).

Q18 The conformation of the ECG waveforms in the thoracic leads indicates:

A. left ventricular hypertrophy
B. left atrial hypertrophy
C. right ventricular hypertrophy
D. right bundle branch block
E. bilateral ventricular hypertrophy

Q19 From your knowledge of the effects of altitude on the circulation, you can deduce that this effect on cardiac function has been triggered by:

A. increased afterload due to polycythaemia
B. increased afterload due to hypoxic vasoconstriction
C. increased afterload due to hypocapnic vasoconstriction
D. ventricular distension secondary to hyperventilation
E. ventricular distension secondary to hypoxia

One of the areas of research at La Oroya is investigation of whether normal adaptations to altitude can enhance competitive athletic performance. As we have seen, the characteristic medium- to long-term responses to altitude include polycythaemia and elevated 2,3-DPG. Consider the implications of these changes for oxygen carriage and exercise capacity.

Q20 In an untrained individual acclimatized to high altitude, you would expect exercise capacity to be:

A. enhanced only at high altitude
B. enhanced at all altitudes but more so at high altitude
C. enhanced at all altitudes but more so at low altitude
D. enhanced equally at all altitudes
E. enhanced at high altitude but reduced at low altitude

Q21 Which of the following would be the best training strategy for athletes to adopt in order to optimize work capacity?

A. live at high altitude and train at low altitude
B. live at low altitude and train at high altitude
C. live and train at high altitude
D. any of the above
E. either B or C depending on the altitude of the competition

Q22 In a competition at high altitude, for which type of event would prior altitude training confer the *least* benefit?

A. events longer than 10 000 m
B. events longer than 5000 m
C. events longer than 1000 m
D. events shorter than 1000 m
E. events shorter than 400 m

Apart from a variable period of adjustment to the hypoxic environment, the visitors from Ireland experience no health problems. Having an opportunity of surveying the health of the local community around La Oroya, however, they do identify several pathologies that may be related to the altitude. One of these is a high incidence of right cardiac failure, probably linked to the increased right ventricular workload discussed above. Another is an incidence of patent ductus arteriosus that is around 15 times that in Peruvian communities at sea level.

Q23 High altitude would predispose towards the ductus arteriosus remaining open after birth because breathing hypoxic air:

A. increases prostaglandin synthesis by the cells of the ductus wall
B. decreases the normal postnatal fall in pulmonary vascular resistance
C. maintains left atrial pressure at a higher level than right atrial pressure
D. both A and B above
E. none of the above

Goitre is another health problem that they find has a much higher incidence than expected in this high-altitude community.

Q24 What is goitre caused by? Why might this be particularly likely in mountainous regions? What other pathologies would you expect to be associated with goitre in such regions?

Thermoregulation is a universal problem with life at high altitude. Atmospheric temperature decreases by 1°C for every 150 m (500 ft) above sea level, so below-freezing temperatures are the norm. Simultaneously, the lack of atmospheric refraction due to lack of water vapour and pollution means that solar radiation is quite powerful. This leads to the paradox that an individual can feel hot, while having a thermal gradient between body and environment that predisposes to rapid body cooling. We will see shortly how dangerous this situation can be.

During the third week of their visit, the students decide as they are well enough acclimatized to walk to a nearby village some 10 km (6 miles) away and at a slightly lower altitude. When they set off the day is bright and sunny and soon most people have taken off their wind jackets, although the temperature in the shade is −10°C.

For the first 2 hours, the walk is an enjoyable one, but then the weather begins to change, with a strong wind and dense cloud beginning to envelop the mountain. The party decides to climb back to La Oroya, which is around 5 km distant. Some members of the party are now beginning to feel extremely cold although they have replaced their jackets. Several of them would like to rest for a while. However, the group decision is that the deteriorating conditions make it safer to try to make base before visibility becomes too poor.

Q25 Several factors may be contributing to falling body temperatures in the walkers at this stage. Think about the circumstances and then identify which one of the following factors would be *unlikely* to be involved (alternatively, you may decide that they are all likely to be important):

A. depletion of muscle glycogen stores
B. cold-induced vasodilation
C. convective cooling by wind chill
D. depletion of free fatty acid stores
E. all these factors are likely to be important

Kathy is walking more slowly than the others and is complaining that she feels very cold. She does not seem to be interested in keeping up and complains that she feels too tired to continue. She is shivering dramatically, with pronounced movements of her arms.

One of the other students has brought along a flask of a local spirit distilled from cactus. She suggests that drinking some of this will make Kathy feel warmer.

Q26 Consuming ethanol tends to produce a feeling of warmth because it:

A. depresses cerebral cortical perception of temperature
B. increases skin blood flow
C. directly depresses cold-sensitive sensory axons
D. directly stimulates warm-sensitive sensory axons
E. non-specifically depresses sensory transmission in the spinal cord

Q27 This effect is due to:

A. thermoregulatory heat-loss processes in response to metabolic heat production
B. thermoregulatory heat-loss processes in response to hypothalamic thermostat resetting
C. direct relaxation of vascular smooth muscle
D. inhibition of transmitter release from vasoconstrictor axon terminals
E. none of the above

About 30 minutes later, Kathy suddenly collapses. She seems confused and is not shivering as much as before. Her skin is very cold and her pulse rate is 40 beats/min.

Q28 The combination of cerebral impairment and reduced shivering suggests that Kathy's deep body temperature has fallen to around:

A. 36°C
B. 34°C
C. 33°C
D. 30°C
E. 27°C

When handling patients who are hypothermic, you have to consider the physiological effects of cold in order not to further endanger their well-being. One factor to remember is that heat loss is increased greatly by evaporation and convection. The first thing to do is therefore to enclose the patient in dry insulation such as a blanket or even thick newspapers. Kathy is wrapped in an insulated blanket ('space blanket') over her clothing, ensuring that her head and neck are well covered since these are important sources of heat loss.

The next consideration is whether to leave Kathy where she is and send for assistance, or to carry her back to La Oroya. Based on the facts that the weather is continuing to deteriorate and that they are now only about 2 km from home, the decision is to carry her. It will be necessary to improvize a stretcher so she can be kept horizontal or head down, since her baroreflex control of blood pressure is likely to be impaired.

Q29 Baroreflex control of blood pressure is likely to be impaired in a patient with severe hypothermia because hypothermia is associated with:

A. reduced heart rate
B. reduced peripheral nerve conduction
C. impaired cerebral function
D. reduced plasma volume
E. both B and D

At La Oroya, Kathy is admitted to the station clinic. Her core temperature measured by oesophageal thermistor is found to be 33.1°C. She is now fully conscious but is still only shivering intermittently and seems to have no memory of the preceding few hours. Her heart rate is 55 beats/min; her blood pressure is 130/66 mmHg. The treatment team must decide whether to allow her to rewarm spontaneously or to rewarm her actively using one of several available modalities.

Q30 Given the circumstances that have led to Kathy's hypothermic state, which of the following strategies for rewarming would be most appropriate?

A. conductive rewarming by immersion in a hot bath
B. radiative rewarming by blowing hot air onto her skin
C. spontaneous rewarming by insulation in a space blanket
D. either A or B
E. either A or C

Treatment is commenced immediately and Kathy's heart rate, blood pressure and core temperature are monitored continuously. Her body temperature rises steadily and within 4 hours she is normothermic. After an overnight stay in the clinic, she is discharged, but is advised not to undertake extended exercise again during her stay. Although there are usually no after-effects of hypothermia in young, healthy individuals, the fatigue and depletion of energy stores makes a recuperation period advisable.

MCQ ANSWERS AND FEEDBACK

1.B. Post-menopausal and non-ovulating women have similar haematocrits to those in ovulating, pre-menopausal individuals, indicating that neither female steroid profile nor menstrual blood loss is a major factor in the characteristic gender difference. This difference is due primarily to a stimulant effect of testosterone on red cell production. Despite the fact that the normal gender difference is independent of menstrual blood loss, it is clinically important to remember that *excessive* blood loss through menstruation is a relatively common cause of anaemia in young women.

2.C. The suffix 'chromic' comes from the Greek word *chroma*, meaning colour, and refers to the amount of haemoglobin in each cell. The suffix 'cytic' refers to the cell size. Julie's blood contains cells that are both smaller than the usual 78–95 fl and contain substantially less haemoglobin than the normal 27–32 pg/cell.

3.E. Normal haemoglobin contains equal numbers of alpha- and beta-globin chains and linkage of these is essential in order for the molecule to be functional. In beta-thalassaemia, insufficient beta-globin chains are synthesized and the unpaired alpha-globins precipitate, damaging the erythrocyte membrane and causing premature haemolysis. The reduced cellular haemoglobin content (*hypochromia*) and rapid cell turnover results in abnormally large numbers of relatively small (*microcytic*), immature cells. A similar picture is seen with iron deficiency. In pernicious anaemia, by contrast, the erythrocytes are larger than normal (*macrocytic*) because they do not undergo the shrinkage that is part of the normal maturational process.

4.A. When sickling haemoglobin molecules pass through a peripheral capillary bed they become deoxygenated and are exposed to increased osmolality due to release of tissue metabolites into the plasma. Consequently, the erythrocytes in which they reside are temporarily stiffened. This reduces the capacity of cells to glide past each other and to fold up as they pass through capillaries. In consequence, blood viscosity is increased and some regions of the microcirculation may become completely blocked.

The fact that the cells are less easily distorted by mechanical pressure means also that their membranes are more easily damaged, leading to premature haemolysis. This reduced lifespan is probably why the sickle cell gene is common in the West African gene pool. By minimizing the period that is available for the malaria parasite to mature inside red cells, inheritance of the heterozygous sickle cell trait confers some resistance to this infection.

5. Hypoxia will certainly increase the rate at which red cells break down and the resulting anaemia will reduce Carl's capacity to carry oxygen from lungs to tissues. However, a more serious problem is that the increased number of sickled cells under hypoxic conditions will increase the likelihood of their blocking blood flow through some functionally important bed (*infarction*). The high probability of infarcts during hypoxia makes it essential to screen patients from susceptible gene pools for sickle cell trait before general anaesthesia.

6.D. The sites susceptible to infarction will be those at which local hypoxia and hyperosmolality are most pronounced. The single site that best fulfils these requirements is the renal medulla. Most of the oxygen in the renal bloodstream has already been extracted by the tubular cells before blood enters the vasa recta. In addition, the medullary interstitial osmolality is around four-fold higher than in any other organ. This unique combination of factors means that renal medullary infarction with diminished urinary concentrating capacity is common in sickle cell heterozygotes. Infarcts may occur at the other sites listed, but usually only in patients with the homozygous disorder.

7.B. The reflex bronchoconstriction that accompanies whole-body aerobic exercise in some asthmatic individuals is due to activation of sensory vagal axons in the airways mucosa. The normal role of these axons is to induce reflex bronchoconstrictor responses to inhaled irritants, but they are also excited by dehydration. Since the likelihood of dehydration is related to the dryness of the inhaled air, and since air humidity falls with decreased temperature, exercise-induced asthma is most likely to occur in the cold.

8.D. The molecular composition of a mixture cannot be altered by simply changing its volume, so oxygen molecules always contribute 21% of the air regardless of the pressure.

9.C. If we presume that the inspired air is dry, humidification in the upper airways will necessarily reduce Po_2 by around 10 mmHg (1.3 kPa) and dilution by the relatively hypoxic and hypercapnic air left over from the previous breath (that is, the functional residual capacity) will reduce it by a further 40 mmHg (5.3 kPa).

10.A. The central chemoreceptors respond to changes in arterial CO_2 but are insensitive to changes in Pao_2.

11.E. If Kathy increases her minute ventilation without a proportionate increase in metabolic rate, then she will blow off more CO_2 from her lungs. Decreased $PAco_2$ will increase diffusion of CO_2 from plasma to air and consequently lower $Paco_2$. One immediate consequence of this hypocapnia will be to elevate plasma pH, because of the relative deficit of protons created.

12.D. Water and CO_2 react to produce carbonic acid. This and the subsequent dissociation of carbonic acid into protons and bicarbonate are essential for blood transport of CO_2 and regulation of body pH. The reactions can occur in either direction, depending on which set of end-products is in higher concentration, and no enzymatic activity is needed. However, carbonic anhydrase greatly speeds up the reactions. It is therefore not surprising that this enzyme is present in all cells whose normal functions require them to produce bicarbonate.

13.B. The efficacy of carbonic anhydrase inhibition indicates that the symptoms are related to disturbed acid–base balance. During the first 24 hours of ascent to altitude, respiratory alkalosis must be the likely cause of this.

14.A. Normally, the dominant respiratory drive is from central chemoreceptors. These detect cerebral interstitial pH, which is regulated primarily by $Paco_2$. Although hypoxia increases ventilation through activating peripheral chemoreceptors, the effect is limited if simultaneous hypocapnia reduces the concentration of protons in the cerebral interstitium and depresses central chemoreceptor activity. During 24 hours sustained hypocapnia, however, excess interstitial bicarbonate diffuses away into the CSF. So interstitial pH and central chemoreceptor drive return to near-normal values.

15.C. Respiratory water loss is only about 600 ml/day with resting ventilation at sea level, but the volume lost at altitude can be substantial. This is due not only to the increased volume of air moving over the airways mucosa but also to the fact that the inspired air is very dry. Water intake therefore needs to be increased substantially at altitude, but during the acute phase of adaptation people commonly find that they do not feel thirsty. There cannot be any effective stimulation of erythropoiesis within the 24-hour period since Kathy left sea level. Neither of the other options will affect haematocrit.

16.B. Respiratory drive from peripheral hypoxia receptors is no longer antagonized by central chemoreceptor depression and therefore the gas tensions achieved within lung and arterial blood will be closer to those in atmospheric air. Pao_2 will rise and $Paco_2$ will fall. Although acid–base compensation will eventually produce a picture similar to that in answer A, renal compensation takes more than one day and will be slowed further by the additional hypocapnia that is caused by increased ventilation.

17.B. Increased expression of 2,3-DPG occurs over 3–4 days when erythrocytes are exposed to hypoxia. However extreme the hypoxic stimulus, no additional haemoglobin can be made available except through the normal cell formation cycle. This will take weeks to become apparent.

18.C. As leads V_1–V_2 are adjacent to the right ventricle and leads V_5–V_6 are adjacent to the left ventricle, the R wave is normally upright in V_5–V_6 and inverted in V_1–V_2. If this pattern is reversed or if the waves in these leads are bipolar then the amount of muscle in the right ventricle must be greater than normal, relative to the left ventricle.

19.B. Intra-airway hypoxia induces both airway dilation and vasoconstriction of neighbouring pulmonary arterioles. This is a useful way of ensuring that ventilation and perfusion are matched optimally in regions of the lung that are inflated to different extents. When all the airways are exposed to a hypoxic gas mixture, however, there is generalized pulmonary vasoconstriction which raises right ventricular afterload. If this persists for many months, the result is right ventricular hypertrophy. The polycythaemia induced by chronic hypoxia will also cause some increase in cardiac afterload but the effect will be similar for right and left ventricles.

20.C. Without doubt, optimal capacity for physical activity at high altitudes relies on prior acclimation so as to improve blood delivery of oxygen. However, under conditions where alveolar Po_2 is less than around 80 mmHg (10.7 kPa), the rightwards shift of the haemoglobin curve induced by 2,3-DPG means that efficiency of pulmonary uploading of oxygen is reduced as well as the offloading in systemic capillaries being improved. At sea level there is no effect on uploading, so the beneficial effect of 2,3-DPG is somewhat greater.

21.A. When athletes train at altitude, the potentially beneficial effects of chronic hypoxia on oxygen carriage capacity are reduced by the lower training intensity that results from reduced air density and oxygen limitation. Better results are obtained by spending around 50% of the day in a hypoxic environment but training at low altitude.

22.E. Sprint performance relies mainly on anaerobic metabolism and therefore track performance over short distances is little affected by the efficiency of oxygen delivery except at very high altitude. In fact, as there is some reduction in air resistance due to the low air density, performance at sprint distances may actually rise. At the Mexico City Olympic Games (2200 m, 7200 ft), records were broken in several sprint events but not in any longer races.

23.D. Prior to birth, the ductus arteriosus is held open by continual secretion of prostaglandins of the E type. Prostaglandin synthesis in the ductus cells is able to occur only under relatively hypoxic conditions. At birth, the onset of respiratory function elevates the absolute oxygen tension in left heart blood, while the accompanying fall in pulmonary vascular resistance reverses the direction of ductus blood flow from right → left to left → right. The resulting increased oxygenation of the ductus cells shuts off prostaglandin production and the ductus constricts.

24. Goitre is hypertrophy of the thyroid gland, secondary to excessive activation of thyroid-stimulating hormone (TSH) receptors. This can be caused by autoimmune stimulation of the receptors, under which circumstances it leads to excessive release of thyroid hormone and thyrotoxicosis (*Graves' disease*). More dramatic hypertrophy is associated, however, with conditions that reduce thyroid hormone production. This prevents feedback inhibition of the anterior pituitary, resulting in extremely high TSH secretion that stimulates massive overgrowth of the follicular cells.

The most common cause of this hypothyroid state is inadequate dietary intake of iodine. Iodine deficiency is particularly common in mountainous regions because the original iodine-rich soil has been washed away by glacial thawing and replaced by new soil derived from iodine-poor rocks. In these areas thyroid hormone production is substantially below normal despite the glandular hypertrophy, resulting in a high incidence of hypothyroidism (*myxoedema*). Hypothyroid dwarfism (*cretinism*) is also common, due to lack of the normal prenatal trophic influence of thyroxine on central nervous system development.

25.D. During demanding exercise, the cerebral depression engendered by mild hypothermia is coupled with depletion of glycogen stores. This induces feelings of fatigue and reduces the amount of metabolic heat produced by the exercise. Ambient temperatures close to or below 0°C cause opening of arteriovenous shunt vessels in small volume : surface area tissues such as digits, ears and nose, and large volumes of blood are directed through these. The shunt flow can be a valuable mechanism to prevent tissue freezing, but simultaneously causes significant heat loss into the environment. As maintenance of normal core temperature depends on adequate insulation of the body core from the environment, exposure of the body surface to convective currents such as wind significantly impairs thermoregulatory capacity.

The listed response that is *least* likely to make a significant contribution to initial fall in body temperature under the conditions indicated is free fatty acid depletion. The small skeletal muscle contractions that are seen as shivering utilize mainly free fatty acids and these persist until body temperature is considerably below normal.

26.B. Increased plasma levels of ethanol produce vasodilation of cutaneous arterioles, with increased skin blood flow and local warming. This causes reduced discharge in cutaneous cold-receptive axons, which will be detected by the brain as a feeling of whole-body warmth regardless of the actual core temperature. At high altitudes, the intense solar radiation often tends to enhance further the perception of warming induced by alcohol ingestion. Since the true ambient temperature is usually well below freezing point, this combination of misleading signals from the skin can easily result in significant body cooling, even in somebody who is not already hypothermic.

27.C. At the plasma levels that are typical of social ingestion, ethanol both relaxes vascular smooth muscle cells and inhibits tonic discharge in the descending spinal neurons responsible for sympathetic vasoconstrictor tone. At very high (toxic) plasma levels, ethanol appears to enhance neurotransmitter release, probably by increasing membrane fluidity.

28.C. Higher mental functions such as reasoning and memory can begin to become impaired at deep body temperatures as high as 35°C, but overt confusion becomes apparent at around 33°C and consciousness is lost over the range of 29–32°C. Other changes that may be helpful in assessing probable core temperature in hypothermic patients are loss of shivering (around 33°C) and cardiac arrest (25–27°C). These values are general guidelines but the absolute temperatures at which any one change occurs varies considerably between patients, dependent mainly on the time course over which hypothermia has developed.

29.B. Since action potential conduction velocity and neural transduction processes are both extremely temperature-dependent, all reflexes involving peripheral nerves become less efficient as body temperature falls. Because peripheral tissue temperatures fall more rapidly than that of the brain, peripheral nerve function can be impaired when cerebral function is still normal. Individuals who have been exposed for prolonged periods to a cold environment will be volume-depleted as well as hypothermic. In such cases, the capacity to maintain cardiac output will be impaired by reduced cardiac filling, but this is independent of the direct effects of low body temperature.

30.A. Individuals who have become moderately hypothermic (that is, who are still conscious and shivering) fairly quickly will usually rewarm spontaneously. In situations where cooling has occurred over an extended period, on the other hand, depletion of energy stores is likely to have occurred – in Kathy's case both through fatiguing exercise and because of shivering. In such circumstances, active rewarming is the preferred option.

Due to the different conductive indices, heat absorption by the body from a liquid environment is far more efficient than that from air. Attempting to rewarm using radiant heat has an additional potential problem associated with it. As soon as the skin is warmed, sensory drive from skin cold receptors to the thermoregulatory centre is turned off, resulting in withdrawal of cutaneous vasoconstrictor tone and a large increase in blood flow to the limbs. Because the underlying tissues of the limbs are still cold, the increased blood flow leads to further heat loss out of the circulation and a net fall in core temperature. This fall can be as great as 2–3°C, which may be sufficient to impair consciousness and complicate recovery.

CASE REVIEW

The adaptive physiology of normal subjects at altitude has provided many insights into clinical conditions such as chronic obstructive lung disease.

Reducing the partial pressure of oxygen has no discernible effect until arterial Po_2 is around 60 mmHg (8.0 kPa) or less, as that is the threshold for activation of peripheral chemoreceptors. A Po_2 of 60 mmHg corresponds to around 3000 m (10 000 ft) so lower altitudes do not usually produce overt hyperventilation or alkalosis, but they can limit exercise capacity because of the slight reduction in haemoglobin saturation.

The pressure inside passenger aircraft corresponds to an altitude around 2400 m (8000 ft). Oxygen availability to air travellers at rest is therefore near normal, although there is evidence that complex mental function is impaired somewhat by even this small degree of hypoxia. In practice, however, potential effects of the aircraft environment on cardiovascular function are of more concern. Passengers easily become dehydrated because of the low humidity, resulting in haemoconcentration. Also, reduced atmospheric pressure on the skin and seated immobility cause peripheral venous pooling. Both factors increase the potential for formation of thrombi in the deep veins of the legs (see Chapter 4).

Rapid ascent to altitudes greater than about 3000 m (10 000 ft) causes the syndrome known as acute mountain sickness in a sizable proportion of normal people. The pathophysiology of this syndrome is complex and not fully understood. There is no doubt that inhibition of carbonic anhydrase prior to ascent reduces symptoms. This treatment works at least partly because the resulting acidosis helps prevent hypocapnic respiratory alkalosis. In addition, however, severe arterial hypoxia causes cerebral arteriolar vasodilatation. The resulting increase in cerebral capillary hydrostatic pressure and consequent cerebral oedema may also contribute to the symptoms of acute mountain sickness. At very high altitudes, therefore, some alleviation of symptoms by carbonic anhydrase inhibition might be due to the diuretic effect that accompanies increased urinary bicarbonate excretion, leading to plasma volume reduction and hence to a fall in cerebral capillary pressure.

There is a dramatic degree of chronic adaptation to altitude, as illustrated by remembering that a number of ascents of Mt Everest have now been carried out without supplementary oxygen. The summit of Mt Everest is 8848 m (29 000 ft) and at this altitude barometric pressure is 253 mmHg (33.7 kPa), so atmospheric Po_2 is 53 mmHg (7.1 kPa) and airways humidification must reduce this to 43 mmHg (5.7 kPa) in the lungs, even without any dilution by intrapulmonary gas. If alveolar Pco_2 were the normal 40 mmHg (5.4 kPa), arterial Po_2 would therefore be zero. Survival at this altitude is only possible if alveolar Pco_2 can be lowered to 10 mmHg (1.3 kPa) or less, which requires a continuous minute ventilation of around 25 litres/min at rest!

The situation discussed in this chapter focuses on short-term adaptation to moderate altitudes. However, many millions of people live permanently at these and higher altitudes in South America and Central Asia. The highest documented permanent settlement is at Tada in Nepal (5770 m, 19 000 ft). At such heights, pronounced degrees of adaptation are seen, including haematocrits up to 70%. The large rise in cardiac workload that results from this, and from the pulmonary vasoconstrictor effect of hypoxia, leads to considerable cardiac hypertrophy and a high frequency of right heart failure in these populations.

The problem of hypothermia is illustrated most graphically with outdoor activities, as set out in this chapter. For urban medical practitioners in the Western world, however, hypothermia is more commonly seen indoors, predominantly in elderly individuals with low incomes. Here, lack of heating and poor nutritional status combine to produce a very slow but progressive fall in body temperature. These patients also typically have impaired baroreflex control, partly because ageing reduces autonomic reflex gain and partly because of reduced plasma volume. This results from the normal cutaneous vasoconstrictor response to cold redirecting an additional proportion of cardiac output to the kidneys, with a proportionate increase in glomerular filtration.

The presence of hypothermia is sometimes self-evident as, for example, with somebody who is rescued from cold water. In other cases, however, it can be difficult to recognize or to confirm. For one thing, clinical thermometers do not record temperatures below around 35°C. Thus, objective evaluation of core temperature may not be possible unless you have a thermometer especially designed for low temperatures. Furthermore, cutaneous vasoconstriction and the counter-current exchange of heat between deep limb arteries and veins means that the extremities are often just as cold in a normothermic individual who has been exposed to cold as in someone with true hypothermia.

Deciding on how to treat hypothermia must take into account both the severity and the cause. After rapid cooling, moderate hypothermia will be reversed by normal metabolic heat production, provided that the patient is well insulated in blankets and wind-resistant wraps. On the other hand, individuals who have been exposed for so long that their metabolic energy stores are depleted will not be able to produce sufficient body heat to rewarm spontaneously.

In these patients and in anyone whose temperature has fallen so far that consciousness is impaired, active rewarming is essential. The warm water immersion approach as indicated in this chapter is quick and effective, but is difficult with an unconscious patient. In the field, hot water packs or the body heat of another person could be used. In regions where cold exposure is frequent, specialized facilities for ventilation with moist, warmed air or intraperitoneal dialysis with warm fluid may be available.

The first essential, however, remains provision of adequate insulation to prevent heat loss. Without this, it is unlikely that any modality for adding heat to the body will be effective in restoring core temperature to normal.

KEY POINTS

- Reduction in alveolar Po_2 to 60 mmHg (8.0 kPa) or less increases minute ventilation by activating peripheral chemoreceptors.
- This hypoxic respiratory drive is limited by the concomitant hypocapnia which depresses central chemoreceptor activity.
- The combination of hypoxia and hypocapnia may lead to central nervous symptoms collectively termed acute mountain sickness.
- Continued exposure to hypoxia results in a variety of adaptive responses that produce dramatic improvement in peripheral oxygen delivery.
- Hypothermia can occur extremely rapidly when perceptions of cold are masked by withdrawal of signals from skin cold receptors.
- Procedures for reversing hypothermia must take account of a variety of normal physiological responses to cold.

ADDITIONAL READING

Basnyat B & Murdoch DR (2003) High-altitude illness. *Lancet* **361**: 1967–74.

Hendriksenn IJ & Meeuwsen T (2003) The effect of intermittent training in hypobaric hypoxia on sea-level exercise: a cross-over study in humans. *European Journal of Applied Physiology* **88**: 396–403.

Sallis R & Chassay CM (1999) Recognizing and treating common cold-induced injury in outdoor sports. *Medicine and Science in Sports and Exercise* **31**: 1367–73.

Schmidt W, Heinicke K, Rojas J *et al.* (2002) Blood volume and hemoglobin mass in endurance athletes from moderate altitude. *Medicine and Science in Sports and Exercise* **34**: 1934–40.

Ward MP, Milledge JS & West JB (2000) *High Altitude Medicine and Physiology*, 3rd edition. Arnold, London.

Two cases of chronic fatigue

CASES AND MCQS

Case 1 introduction

A 44-year-old male, Mr R.McD., who had previously been an executive producer with a television company, has had a difficult period over the past 10 years or so. Early in his career he was a lively, energetic and creative individual who got on well with people. His career and personal relationships developed well and he and his partner had a child. However, he progressively became somewhat lethargic; he became disinterested and detached from his family and friends: eventually he and his partner separated.

Subsequently, his eyes began to feel 'puffy' and he had occasional pains in the chest. He thought this might be due to 'burning the candle at both ends'. Despite having a small appetite he put on weight. Eventually he also had to resign his job. He felt that he was suffering from the pressure of the work and thought that he was suffering from work-related depression.

He talked with his GP who gave him antidepressant tablets and told him to 'take things easy'. The tablets helped somewhat but he still did not regain his physical or creative energies. Earlier in life he had played football regularly and did a lot of running; he now found that he very rapidly became fatigued and tired and as a consequence he gave up all forms of exercise. Recently, friends have told him that his voice has changed and become lower and husky. He suffers badly in the winter with the cold and at the end of a day his shoes feel tight.

Friends and colleagues have also told him that his personality has changed greatly. In the past, he had been energetic, lively and 'great fun' whereas he is now very lethargic and had become much less interesting as a person. He writes poetry and friends have also told him that when reading poetry or novels aloud his speech is slurred and without its usual lively character. He has been aware of some of these changes but had put them down to the depression and the fact that he was older! However, the comments of his friends have now stimulated him to approach a doctor again.

You spend some considerable time talking with Mr McD. before examining him. He recounts his past history and says that he still feels depressed. He is clearly very lethargic and intolerant of moderate exercise. When he goes on short walks, muscle pain and fatigue quickly develop in his legs and he has to stop. He does not like the cold weather at all. He has suffered from constipation for many years and uses laxatives to relieve it. You find that he is mentally quite slow, finding it difficult to do simple calculations or to make a logical set of deductions. His intellectual performance is clearly well below that which he had previously been capable of and exercised in his job.

Physical examination shows an individual who is quite portly for his age. The skin of his arms and legs is pale, coarse and dry. His hair is thin and coarse, his face is pale and round and his lower eyelids are puffy (Fig. 15.1). His speech is slow and slurred.

His blood pressure is high normal (137/87 mmHg) and his heart rate is low (55 beats/min). There are some signs of oedema in his legs; thus his socks are tight and leave marks on his lower legs. However, there is no evidence that jugular venous pressure is elevated. His breathing is slow and steady and his mucous membranes are pale pink.

He tells you that, at times, his finger joints seem to be thick and he finds it difficult to coordinate his fingers to carry out precise tasks.

On the basis of his history and symptoms, one possibility is that he may be suffering from cardiac or renal disease.

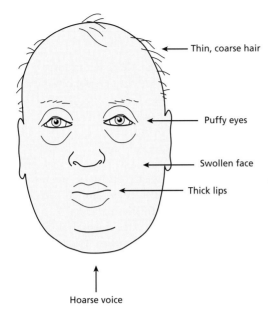

Thin, coarse hair

Puffy eyes

Swollen face

Thick lips

Hoarse voice

Fig. 15.1 Patient R.McD. at time of his first visit to you.

Q1 Which of his symptoms are consistent with a renal or cardiac problem?

A. fatigue on exercise
B. peripheral oedema
C. facial oedema
D. pain in the chest
E. all of the above

A chest X-ray reveals no signs of pulmonary oedema or enlargement of the heart. An ECG is essentially normal and shows only low voltage P and T waves with a slight prolongation of the QT interval. His 24-hour urinary volumes and tonicities are within normal limits. A venous blood sample is taken for biochemistry and the relevant results are listed below:

Total cholesterol	6.2 mmol/l
HDL cholesterol	1.0 mmol/l
LDL cholesterol	3.8 mmol/l
Sodium	135 mmol/l
Potassium	4.6 mmol/l
Red cell count	4.0×10^{12}/l
Haemoglobin	12.0 g/dl

Q2 These data indicate:

A. all listed values are normal
B. anaemia
C. anaemia and hyponatraemia
D. anaemia, hyponatraemia and hypercholesterolaemia
E. hypokalaemia and hypercholesterolaemia

The report also shows that plasma creatinine phosphokinase and lactic dehydrogenase are slightly elevated. All other variables are normal.

You conclude that Mr McD. is not suffering from renal or cardiac disease.

Q3 Briefly summarize the important findings and observations that lead to this conclusion.

At this stage, let us list the various symptoms that have been identified. All may be important indicators towards an eventual diagnosis.

- Progressive development of lethargy and lack of interest in other people.
- Decline in intellectual performance.
- Change in voice and lack of verbal expression.
- Slight peripheral oedema and constipation.
- Puffy eyes.
- Inability to cope with physical exercise and cold.

You carry out a short examination of Mr McD.'s peripheral neuromuscular function. The salient results are:

- There is clear evidence of weakness of the proximal skeletal muscles.
- Some evidence of carpal tunnel syndrome is present.
- Examination of peripheral reflexes shows that there is very slow relaxation of the muscle following elicitation of ankle jerks on each side.

A further venous blood sample is taken and radio-immune hormone assays are performed.

Q4 Given the evidence above, which hormones should be assayed?

A. thyroid hormone and growth hormone
B. thyroid hormone and thyroid-stimulating hormone
C. thyroid-stimulating hormone and growth hormone
D. growth hormone and growth hormone-releasing factor
E. growth hormone and cortisol

The assay results are:

Thyroid hormone (T_3 and T_4)	T_3 <0.1 nmol/l; T_4 <10 nmol/l (normal T_3 0.9–28 nmol/l; T_4 50–150 nmol/l)
Thyroid-stimulating hormone (TSH)	110 mIU/l (normal 20 mIU/l)
Thyroid-binding globulin (TBG)	0.1 μmol/l (normal 0.3 μmol/l)
Albumin	636 μmol/l (normal 640 μmol/l)

You decide that Mr McD. is suffering from a deficiency of thyroid hormone (*hypothyroidism*).

Q5 What are the crucial new pieces of evidence used for the diagnosis?

A. low thyroid hormone
B. high TSH
C. delayed ankle jerks
D. lethargy and impaired mental state
E. all of the above

Q6 TSH is elevated because of:

A. lack of feedback inhibition of the hypothalamus
B. lack of feedback inhibition of the anterior pituitary gland
C. lack of dietary iodine
D. lack of physical activity
E. none of the above

The treatment for hypothyroidism consists of oral thyroxine (100–200 μg/day) for life. The dose is adjusted over several months to match the patient's requirements.

Mr McD. recovers his health and mental abilities very quickly and has now resumed his creative role in the media and writing.

Case 2 introduction

A 30-year-old woman, Mrs M.C., complains of feeling very tired when walking home from the local shops, especially when she is carrying shopping bags. She had been very keen on tennis and used to play several times a week; but now she finds it impossible as, very quickly after starting a game, she becomes very fatigued and her strokes seem to have no power.

Recently, at home in the evenings, she has had several episodes of double vision (*diplopia*) but did not notice any-thing that might have triggered this. She also notices that, at the end of a day, her eyelids tend to droop (*ptosis*). When she smiles, her facial muscles do not maintain their con-traction; this introduces a progressive 'snarling' appearance. Not unexpectedly, she is very upset at these very recent de-velopments.

She also says that she has been finding it difficult to chew her food properly, as her jaw muscles become fatigued.

On examination, she appears a normal healthy woman, both lively and attractive. She has normal blood pressure (120/75 mmHg) and heart rate (70 beats/min) and chest ex-amination reveals nothing unusual about her heart or lungs.

You test her peripheral somatic reflexes.

Q1 What are the somatic reflexes that can be readily tested?

All of Mrs C.'s reflexes appear to be normal. However, when you test her ability to clench her fists she is only able to main-tain this for a very short time. Further, when you test the strength of the muscles in her arms and shoulders by asking her to bend her arm against counter-force that you exert on her hand and wrist, she is clearly very weak. She is also unable to sustain contractions of her arm muscles for a significant period of time. Otherwise, her musculoskeletal system ap-pears normal and there is no muscle wasting.

You then test her ability to control the movements of her eyeballs by asking her to gaze upwards for about 40 s. She

finds this difficult and her ptosis becomes much worse as the period of looking upward progresses.

Muscle weakness can be a symptom of diabetes and of rheu-matoid arthritis; in the case of arthritis, it can be triggered by the drug D-penicillamine that is used to treat the condition. Howev-er, in the present case, the patient's history confirms that she is not suffering from either diabetes mellitus or rheumatoid arthritis.

Q2 What are your thoughts on the most significant symptoms so far?

Q3 What are the common features of these symptoms?

At this stage, it will be useful to review your knowledge of the basis of skeletal muscle contraction under physiological conditions.

In the spinal cord, the alpha-motoneurons initiate contrac-tion via action potentials in the motor nerve fibres passing to the muscles. The motoneurons in the spinal cord fire asynchronously at relatively low frequencies and each impulse is discretely transmitted in the nerve, the neuromuscular junction and the evoked electrical responses in the muscle fibres (muscle action potentials).

In the muscle itself, summation of individual contractions at the contractile machinery level induces a smooth development of force in the muscle that is graded depending on the frequency of firing and the number of motor units activated. Refresh your memory of what constitutes a motor unit. Later, we will discuss some of the fine detail within this cascade of events.

Q4 A motor unit is:

A. the skeletal muscle fibres that are contracting at any one time
B. the skeletal muscle fibres innervated by a single motoneuron
C. the minimum number of muscle fibres needed to cause a change in muscle length when activated
D. a motoneuron and the skeletal muscle fibres innervated by that neuron
E. none of the above

Q5 During contractions in skeletal muscle the:

A. muscle action potentials summate
B. force of contraction varies with the frequency and number of muscle action potentials
C. muscle twitches summate to increase the force developed
D. none of the above
E. both B and C above

You refer Mrs C. to a neurology clinic for tests of her peripheral nerve function.

It will be useful at this point to refresh your knowledge of the different types of peripheral nerve fibres, their roles and their conduction velocities. The motor (*efferent*) and sensory (*afferent*) axons in a peripheral nerve are of several types depending on their diameter and their myelination: all will be stimulated by an electrical stimulus to the whole nerve, producing conduction of impulses in both directions.

Q6 Conduction velocity in an axon is increased by:

A. decreased diameter of the axon
B. myelination of the axon
C. increased amplitude of the action potential
D. the axon being sensory in function
E. all of the above

Q7 Saltatory conduction in axons is:

A. characteristic only of myelinated axons
B. characteristic only of nonmyelinated axons
C. responsible for one-way conduction along axons
D. characteristic only of motor axons
E. none of the above

Q8 The compound action potential that is recorded extracellularly from a nerve has a complex form with several peaks, as shown in Fig. 15.2. What are these due to?

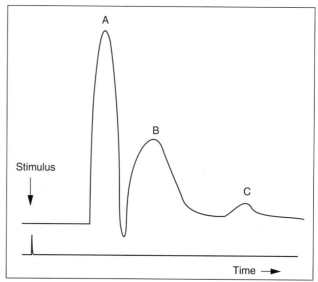

Fig. 15.2 An extracellular recording from a peripheral nerve trunk, showing the three main peaks (A, B and C) that occur at different times after a single electrical stimulation.

The results of Mrs C.'s tests are as follows:

- Recordings of the compound action potentials in her radial and ulnar nerves indicate that conduction is normal in both nerves and that the conduction velocities are within normal limits.
- Repetitive nerve stimulation at supramaximal voltage and 5–10 Hz and recordings of skeletal muscle force and action potential electromyogram (EMG) show, first, that the amplitude of contractions decline progressively and rapidly and, secondly, that the EMG declines in parallel.
- Recordings of skeletal muscle electrical activity and contractions following single and repetitive direct stimulation of the calf and thigh muscles indicate that both contractile force and EMG are maintained during repetitive electrical stimulation.

Q9 The combined results of the nerve stimulation tests and recordings of resultant muscle contraction indicate:

A. failure of nerve conduction
B. failure of transmission at the nerve–muscle interface
C. failure of transmitter breakdown at the nerve–muscle interface
D. failure of the muscle action potential
E. failure of the muscle contractile apparatus

Here we have a disturbance that is characterized by an inability to sustain skeletal muscular effort. Before developing this conclusion we should briefly review some of the detailed mechanisms of neuromuscular transmission at the motor nerve endplate.

An action potential in the motor axon invades the motor endplate – you may wish to check the structure of the endplate itself in a textbook – and causes an influx of calcium ions into the axon terminal. This mobilizes the vesicles in the terminal so that they migrate to the pre-junctional membrane and release their contents, acetylcholine molecules, into the synaptic cleft. The release is thus in the form of packets, or quanta, each of which comprises approximately 100 molecules of acetylcholine. After diffusing across the cleft the acetylcholine stimulates nicotinic acetylcholine receptors on the muscle membrane. This induces a local endplate potential in the muscle fibres, which in turn evokes a muscle action potential, which in turn causes a contraction.

Normally, the number of vesicles released and the amount of acetylcholine available is enough to excite every muscle fibre in response to every action potential; that is, there is a large 'safety factor' for transmission. However, this safety margin could be reduced by either defective synthesis or release of acetylcholine or by inactivation of the post-junctional receptors.

You give Mrs C. an intravenous injection of edrophonium (Tensilon), a short-lasting anticholinesterase. This transiently improves the weakness in her forearm muscles and her ability to smile properly, but the effects last only 1–3 minutes.

Q10 Reduction of motor symptoms after inhibition of acetylcholinesterase is consistent with the patient's problems being due to:

A. reduced neural release of acetylcholine
B. reduced neural synthesis of acetylcholine
C. reduced post-junctional nicotinic acetylcholine receptors
D. any of the above
E. none of the above

From the spectrum of symptoms and the clinical investigations carried out, you conclude that Mrs C. is suffering from myasthenia gravis. This is a disorder that is characterized by a reduced number of receptor sites on the muscle membrane available to respond to acetylcholine.

The symptomatic treatment is to increase the concentration of acetylcholine in the junctional cleft by oral administration of a long-lasting anticholinesterase drug such as pyridostigmine. The duration of even the longest-acting drug of this type is only around 6 hours, so it will be necessary for Mrs C. to take several doses each day if she is to retain a reasonably constant level of motor capacity. As well, emotional and physical status, infections and menstruation all reduce the potency of these agents and may necessitate increased administration frequency or dosage. Careful clinical monitoring of the patient will therefore be essential.

CASE 1 MCQ ANSWERS AND FEEDBACK

1.E. All of these alternatives *may* be associated with cardiac or renal disease.

2.B. Normal red cell values for an adult man are 4.5–6.0×10^{12} cells/l and 13.0–17.0 g haemoglobin/dl. Normal plasma sodium is 135–145 mmol/l. Desirable plasma lipid levels are HDL >0.9 mmol/l, LDL <4.9 mmol/l, total cholesterol <6.0 mmol/l (ideally <5.2 mmol/l).

3. There is no evidence that central venous pressure is elevated – this is very important in discounting cardiac failure as a reason for the oedema. The oedema and occasional chest pain are at relatively low levels. The blood chemistry gives only weak evidence of potential atheroma. The blood electrolytes are not indicative of a major disturbance to renal function. The presence of other symptoms is also important. The coarse, dry, pale skin, puffy eyelids and round face, the slow and slurred gruff speech and difficulty in completing fine movements all suggest some condition that is independent of the cardiovascular or renal systems.

4.B. Nothing in the history suggests that this patient has an abnormality related to growth hormone or to adrenocorticoid activity. His signs and symptoms are compatible with reduced metabolic rate, indicating that it would be useful to know the plasma levels of T_3 (tri-iodothyronine) and T_4 (thyroxine), TBG (thyroxine-binding globulin), TSH (thyroid-stimulating hormone) and albumin. Both TBG and albumin bind appreciable amounts of thyroid hormones (TBG 75% of T_3 and T_4, albumin 15% of T_4 and 0.3% T_3).

5.E. All these are characteristic findings in hypothyroid states.

6.B. TSH levels are normally determined by the levels of circulating thyroid hormone in the blood passing to the anterior pituitary gland. An increase in thyroid hormone induces decreased levels of TSH (Fig. 15.3). If no thyroid hormone is being secreted then the negative feedback loop on the system is broken and an increase in TSH results.

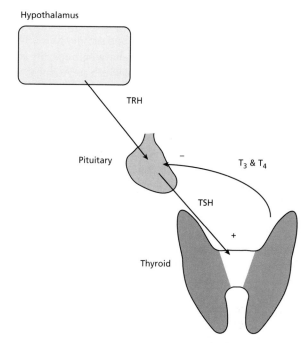

Fig. 15.3 Control of thyroid hormone secretion, showing the negative (–) feedback of secreted thyroxine and tri-iodothyronine on pituitary release of thyroid-stimulating hormone (TSH). Note that, by contrast with some other endocrine feedback loops, there is no feedback from the final hormone onto hypothalamic releasing-factor secretion.

CASE 2 MCQ ANSWERS AND FEEDBACK

1. Knee jerk, ankle jerk, biceps jerk, triceps jerk, supinator jerk, plantar reflex, lower jaw reflex, nasopalpebral (glabellar) reflex, reflex withdrawal to noxious stimulus.

2/3. The weakness and inability to sustain arm skeletal muscle contractions (note the tennis problems in her history as well as your tests in the surgery), drooping of eyelids and inability to maintain upward gaze for a sustained period, and weakness of facial muscles that affects smiling are all characteristic of abnormal skeletal muscle function. The absence of spasticity and preservation of voluntary control and coordination suggest that the problem is located in the peripheral neuromuscular system. Possible sites are the peripheral motor nerves, the neuromuscular junction or the skeletal muscle itself.

4.D. Excitation of a single motor unit will result in contraction only of the muscle fibres supplied by that neuron.

5.E. The force of contraction increases as the number of axons activated increases and as the frequency of muscle action po-

tentials is increased. Action potentials are all-or-none events and cannot summate.

6.B. Conduction velocity rises with axonal diameter and is faster in myelinated than in non-myelinated axons of the same diameter, regardless of whether they are sensory or motor in function. Action potential amplitude does not affect how rapidly depolarization spreads along the axon membrane.

7.A. Saltatory conduction is the term that describes impulse conduction in myelinated fibres, where the action potential leaps from one node of Ranvier to the next. In non-myelinated fibres, the velocity of action potential is slower because it must depolarize all regions of the axon membrane.

8. Action potentials travel at different speeds in different axons and therefore those fibres with the highest conduction velocities arrive at the recording electrodes first, with the slower fibres progressively making their contribution later. Each peak of the compound action potential reflects the summed action potentials of a particular axon group – remember that action potentials in individual axons are *all or none*. The categories are:

- *A-fibres*. These are somatic motor and sensory fibres. They include alpha, beta and gamma/delta subgroups, the conduction velocities and diameters of which are A(alpha) 50–120 m/s and 8–20 µm; A(beta) 30–70 m/s and 5–12 µm; A(gamma/delta) 30–10 m/s and 1–8 µm.
- *B-fibres*. These are the autonomic myelinated preganglionic fibres and are unlikely to be present in significant numbers in peripheral somatic nerves. Their conduction velocities are 5–15 m/s and their diameters are 1–3 µm.
- *C-fibres*. These are unmyelinated and are a mix of sensory and autonomic afferent fibres and autonomic post-ganglionic fibres. Their conduction velocities are <2.5 m/s and their diameters <1 µm.

Overall, it can be seen that conduction velocities vary significantly by a factor of 300–400 and this alone is sometimes used as a system of classification for sensory fibres. Both A(gamma/delta)- and B-fibres contribute to the B peak in the compound action potential.

9.B. The results of peripheral nerve stimulation indicate that conduction in the nerves is essentially normal. Equally, the maintained amplitude of muscle contractions and the associated EMG following direct repetitive electrical stimulation of the muscle suggests that there is not a problem with the skeletal muscle itself. The decrementing EMG and contractile responses to repetitive nerve stimulation suggest progressive failure of chemical transmission at the neuromuscular junction. Failure of transmitter inactivation would if anything increase the muscle response to nerve activation.

10.D. The time course of action of acetylcholine is normally only a few milliseconds because it is rapidly destroyed by the enzyme acetylcholinesterase that is present in high concentration on the post-synaptic membrane. This means that receptor activation occurs only once and only at receptors that are close to the release site. Inhibiting the activity of this enzyme will increase the concentration and the persistence of acetylcholine in the neuromuscular cleft. This will increase the likelihood of effective muscle cell depolarization by otherwise insufficient amounts of acetylcholine. It will also increase the chance of transmitter molecules reaching receptors that are some distance away from the release site. This will improve the efficiency of transmission under circumstances where there is an abnormally low density of receptors on the muscle membrane.

CASE REVIEW

Both of these cases involve destruction of tissue function by the patient's own immune system; in the first case the cells of the thyroid gland and in the second case neurotransmitter receptors at the neuromuscular junction.

Normally the presence of a foreign substance provokes specific lymphocytes to produce an antibody that neutralizes or destroys the antigen: this is clearly an important protective mechanism in the body. For reasons that are presently unclear, antibodies are sometimes produced that destroy specific cells and tissues within the host itself – self-destruction. These antibodies clearly have a genetic locus but their control mechanisms are not known. Autoimmune disorders are of two major types: those that attack specific organs and cells (frequently endocrine organs) and those that attack tissues more generally.

Examples of the organ-specific disorders are those that result from attacks on the thyroid (Hashimoto's and Graves' diseases), adrenal, pancreas (destruction of islet cells resulting in diabetes), liver, gut, skin, nerve and muscle (myasthenia gravis). In disorders of the non-organ-specific type the lesions are more generally distributed; for example, autoimmune arthritis of the joints (rheumatoid arthritis) is also associated with lesions in lungs, eyes, skin, heart, muscle and bone. The autoantibodies can usually, but not always, be detected in the blood of patients, although the existence of an antibody does not necessarily mean that this is the causal agent. Autoimmune disorders are often associated with the thymus and with thymic tumours.

The thyroid gland has a profound effect on a wide range of bodily functions. All cells require an exposure to its hormones at some stage. While the general action is the regulation of gene transcription, the resulting effect depends on the tissue. In the thyroid gland, iodine combines with tyrosine attached to thyroglobulin in the follicles. Thyroxine (T_4) is formed in greater quantities than tri-iodothyronine (T_3) but is less active. These hormones can be stored in the thyroid follicles for several months and are transported in the blood attached to albumin and globulin fractions. In the tissues, their main effect is to increase DNA transcription which increases protein synthesis, enzyme production, size and number of mitochondria and cell membrane transport.

In the fetus, the newborn and the young child differentiation and growth of neural skeletal and most tissues is also dependent on adequate exposure to thyroid hormone. Severe deformities, including cretinism, occur as a result of an absence of the hormone in children.

The thyroid seems to be especially prone to autoimmune attack, resulting in hypothyroidism as described in case 1.

This illustrates the typical development of a disease that affects approximately 2–3% of the population, with 5–17% having a milder subclinical hypothyroid state and with about 90% of cases occurring in females. Since several symptoms of hypothyroidism are shared by a variety of other diseases, the definitive test is administration of oral thyroxine. If this removes the symptoms then a hypothyroid state was present.

In adults, the insidious nature of the progression of autoimmune hypothyroidism means that it is frequently not recognized for many years. Patients put their symptoms down to age, obesity or mental state. Metabolic rate is diminished, core temperature is lowered, protein, carbohydrate and lipid metabolism are altered and progressively more severe effects on the central nervous system develop with time.

The overall set of symptoms is termed *myxoedema*. It includes the voice changes, bagginess under the eyes and the swelling of the face that induces the characteristic appearance. The facial swelling can be explained as follows: for currently unknown reasons, an increase in the amount of hyaluronic acid and chondroitin sulphate bound to tissue protein occurs. This is deposited as an excess of tissue gel in the interstitial space, which attracts interstitial fluid, and results in oedema that is, incidentally, non-pitting.

While the case we have dealt with involved destruction of thyroid cells and removal of the normal feedback inhibition of TRH and TSH secretion, hypothyroidism can also arise from failure of hypothalamic TRH synthesis or of pituitary TSH synthesis, or from a dietary intake of iodine that is insufficient to produce normal amounts of thyroid hormone. These different causes can be associated with different physical signs: thus, thyroid gland hypertrophy (*goitre*) frequently accompanies hypothyroidism due to iodine deficiency, but there is no goitre when the defect is due to loss of secretory tissue. Furthermore, goitre is also a characteristic of some types of hyperthyroidism.

Different causes of the hypothyroid condition produce different combinations of plasma T_3/T_4 and TSH levels, so it is important to measure these. Finding of a high plasma TSH level suggests that autoimmune destruction of the thyroid tissue (*Hashimoto's disease*) is the primary cause. The secretion of TSH is under the control of a negative feedback loop from the anterior pituitary that is triggered by the plasma level of thyroid hormone: in the absence of thyroxine secreted by the thyroid gland, this loop is opened and so an excess of TSH is secreted. Further confirmation can be obtained by testing for the presence of specific antibodies and by taking a biopsy of cells from the gland to demonstrate destruction of secretory thyroid tissue.

The converse disease, an excess of thyroid hormone secretion due to autoimmune stimulation of TSH receptors on the thyroid cells, is known as Graves' disease – *thyrotoxicosis* or *hyperthyroidism*. The symptoms in many ways are, as is to be expected, the opposite of those described above and TSH will be low because of feedback inhibition by the high circulating thyroxine level. Table 15.1 lists the salient signs and symptoms of hypo- and hyperthyroidism.

Case 2 is an example of the autoimmune process destroying a specific set of acetylcholine receptors on the muscle membrane within the neuromuscular junction. Serum antibodies against the nicotinic receptor have been detected in over 80% of cases of myasthenia gravis. The antibodies seem to enhance degradation of nicotinic receptors by muscle enzyme systems, with the result that there are fewer receptors available to stimulate muscle contraction.

Table 15.1 Effects of disturbed thyroid function

	Hypothyroid	Hyperthyroid
Appearance		
Goitre	Sometimes present	Present
Behaviour	Cold-intolerant	Heat-intolerant
	Lethargic, low intellectual performance (+ impaired mental development in perinatal period)	Restless, rapid mentation
Metabolism		
Basal metabolic rate	Lowered	Raised
Core temperature	Lowered	Raised
Protein turnover	Decreased	Increased
Appetite	Lowered	Raised
Body mass	Increased	Decreased
Glucose absorption	Decreased	Increased
Cardiovascular system		
Resting heart rate	Low	High
Resting cardiac output	Low	High
Resting blood pressure	Low	High
Plasma lipid profile	High cholesterol	Low cholesterol
Plasma free T_3/T_4	Low/absent	High

Myasthenia gravis affects around 1 in 25 000 of the population, with a prevalence in women that is twice that of men. The disease starts with weakness of the extraocular eye muscles and progresses to bulbar, neck and proximal limb muscles before involving distal muscle groups: the diaphragm can be involved at late stages, with consequent effects on breathing. The sequence of progression can be explained by the size and number of motor units in the muscles. Because excitation of single muscle fibres is blocked in an 'all-or-none' manner, the actions of muscles with different-sized motor units are affected differently. The effects are seen first in the control of the eyeballs because the extrinsic eye muscles have only around 13 muscle fibres per motor unit and last in respiratory muscles which have >2500 fibres per unit. Thus, the progressive development of the disease over the body from distal to proximal muscles may also be related to the variable innervation ratios.

A reduction in receptor numbers could be predicted to cause comparable impairment of muscular responses to a single or to repetitive action potentials, but the patient with myasthenia gravis is characterized by much more severe impairment of sustained than of brief muscle activity. It is likely that the receptors that survive autoimmune attack are abnormal in having prolonged deactivation times after they bind acetylcholine, so that the number that can be utilized declines during repetitive stimulation.

There is an association between myasthenia gravis, thyrotoxicosis and tumours of the thymus, and removal of the thymus can sometimes alleviate the situation. As well, the immune response can be 'damped down' by immunosuppressant drugs such as corticosteroids, which provide some relief.

Another myasthenic condition (Lambert–Eaton syndrome) results from a different defect at the neuromuscular junction that also appears to arise as a result of autoimmune activity. This is a pre-junctional failure of the release of acetylcholine, due to an antibody against the calcium channels that are essential for exocytosis. Because these channels are similar in all cholinergic axon terminals, Lambert–Eaton syndrome has autonomic as well as somatic manifestations.

The processes involved in cholinergic neuromuscular transmission are sensitive to a much wider range of drugs and toxins than affect other synapses and this has substantial clinical implications. As well as being useful in strengthening inefficient transmission as seen in the present case, inhibitors of acetylcholinesterase are used widely as pesticides and so are a relatively common source of poisoning, where the toxic effects are due to overactivity at cholinergic synapses. Tubocurarine and its derivatives block the access of acetylcholine to nicotinic receptors and are widely used to relax skeletal muscle tone during surgery. These curariform agents produce long-lasting neuromuscular blockade. Another class of drugs that inhibit acetylcholine binding, characterized by succinylcholine, cause initial depolarization of the muscle membrane and induce relaxation only after fasciculation. Because the structure of these agents allows them to be broken down by cholinesterase, they have a much shorter timecourse of action than the curariform drugs. Toxins such as botulinum toxin, produced by *Clostridium botulinum*, bind to the pre-synaptic nerve membrane and produce long-lasting inhibition of acetylcholine exocytosis. This action has recently been used in cosmetic surgery to remove wrinkles.

KEY POINTS

- The thyroid gland and the neuromuscular junction are both relatively common targets of autoimmune attack.
- Autoimmune hypothyroid states are characterized by slow mental and physical activities, reduced metabolism and consequent intolerance of cold and physical activity.
- In these patients, there is high plasma TSH and low plasma thyroid hormone.
- The treatment is administration of oral thyroxine for life.
- Autoimmune destruction of nicotinic acetylcholine receptors on skeletal muscle results in the disease termed myasthenia gravis.
- This is characterized by progressive failure of skeletal muscle contraction on repetitive stimulation of the nerve.
- It is commonly manifested as weakness, ptosis and an inability to maintain upward gaze of the eyes.
- Peripheral somatic reflexes and nerve conduction are normal.
- The motor weakness is reversed transiently by administration of an anticholinesterase agent.

ADDITIONAL READING

Griffin S & Ojeda SR (ed.) (2000) *Textbook of Endocrine Physiology*, 4th edition. Oxford University Press, Oxford.

Keesey JC (2004) A history of treatments for myasthenia gravis. *Seminars in Neurology* **24**: 5–16.

Roitt IM (2001) *Essential Immunology*, 10th edition. Blackwell Science, Oxford.

Wilson JD, Forster DW, Kronenburg HM & Larsen PR (1998) *William's Textbook of Endocrinology*, 9th edition. W.B. Saunders, Philadelphia.

A footballer's painful knee

CASE AND MCQS

Case introduction

J.N., age 17, presents at the emergency room of the hospital in his football gear. That afternoon while playing football, he developed severe pain in his right knee. This was not related to any injury but occurred spontaneously while he was running. It prevented him from continuing playing. He has had no previous illnesses, but when young he had a history of bed-wetting that resolved by the age of six. He has been in very good health and has represented his school at football and he hopes to make a career as a professional footballer. Physical examination reveals a fit, healthy, well-muscled youth. He has a painful right knee and this is tender particularly over the middle of the patella, but there is no degree of swelling.

Blood pressure is 165/97 mmHg, pulse rate is 60 beats/min. His conjunctivae appear to be slightly pale.

X-ray of the knee reveals a stress fracture of the patella and other radiological changes in the bones. Blood analysis shows:

Haemoglobin	10.5 g/dl
Haematocrit	33% (0.33)
Normochromic normocytic anaemia	
Normal white cell count	
Plasma creatinine	0.25 mmol/l (normal 0.06–0.12)
Plasma urea	15.8 mmol/l (normal 2.5–8)

The elevated plasma creatinine and elevated urea indicates that this patient has renal failure. Urine testing reveals no protein, no blood and normal microscopy. There is no family history of renal disease.

Q1 Which of the following is the most likely cause of J.N.'s elevated serum creatinine? (Do not worry if you don't know the answer to this at this time.)

A. polycystic kidneys
B. glomerulonephritis
C. nephrotic syndrome
D. reflux nephropathy
E. renal artery stenosis

Q2 J.N. has (a) high blood pressure; (b) normochromic normocytic anaemia and (c) a stress fracture of the patella. Which of these would be likely consequences of chronic renal disease?

A. (a)
B. (a) and (b)
C. (b) and (c)
D. (a) and (c)
E. (a), (b) and (c)

Q3 Which one of the following blood chemistry profiles is the most likely finding in a person with early chronic renal failure?

A. pH normal; K^+ normal; HCO_3^- low; Ca^{2+} normal
B. pH low; K^+ normal; HCO_3^- low; Ca^{2+} normal
C. pH normal; K^+ normal; HCO_3^- normal; Ca^{2+} low
D. pH low; K^+ elevated; HCO_3^- low; Ca^{2+} low
E. pH low; K^+ normal; HCO_3^- normal; Ca^{2+} low

Q4 In patients with renal failure, there is an increased risk of bone fractures. On a mechanistic basis, which one of the following is the most likely trigger for the development of bone disease in such patients?

A. high parathyroid hormone
B. low plasma phosphate
C. high plasma phosphate
D. low plasma calcium
E. high plasma calcium

Q5 If we measured a number of plasma markers related to calcium in J.N. at his initial presentation, which of the following would *not* be found?

A. normal vitamin D (cholecalciferol)
B. low 25-hydroxyvitamin D
C. low 1,25-dihydroxyvitamin D
D. high parathyroid hormone
E. high serum phosphate

Q6 Which of the following is J.N. most likely to have?

A. low serum calcium
B. high serum sodium
C. high serum potassium
D. high plasma renin
E. high plasma parathyroid hormone

Answer questions 7 to 11 using the five causes of secondary (= *non-essential*) hypertension listed below.

A. bilateral adrenal hyperplasia
B. adrenocortical tumour
C. renal artery stenosis
D. pheochromocytoma
E. renin-secreting tumour

Q7 Which one of these is the most common cause of secondary hypertension?

Q8 Which one of these is most likely to be associated with the combination of high renin, high aldosterone, low plasma potassium, severe hypertension?

Q9 Which one of these is most likely to be associated with the combination of low renin, high aldosterone, low plasma potassium, moderate hypertension?

Q10 Which one of these is most likely to be associated with the combination of low or normal renin, normal plasma potassium, episodic severe hypertension?

Q11 Which one of these is most likely to be associated with the combination of low renin, low plasma potassium, abnormal glucose, abdominal striae, moderate to severe hypertension?

Q12 In the case of patient J.N., his elevated blood pressure is most likely to be due to:

A. sodium retention due to renal failure
B. increased angiotensin II due to excess renin secretion
C. elevated aldosterone
D. essential hypertension
E. increased cardiac output

Q13 If J.N.'s renal function had been investigated 5 years ago when his glomerular filtration rate (GFR) was 60 ml/min, which of the following parameters would have been most likely to be abnormal?

A. urinary concentrating ability
B. urinary diluting ability
C. serum creatinine
D. serum urea
E. plasma aldosterone

Further investigations reveal the following plasma electrolytes:

Sodium	138 mmol/l
Potassium	4.7 mmol/l
Chloride	108 mmol/l
Bicarbonate	18 mmol/l
Calcium	2.24 mmol/l
Phosphate	1.95 mmol/l
Urea	15.8 mmol/l
Creatinine	0.25 mmol/l
pH	7.31

- Bone X-rays show evidence of renal osteodystrophy with elements of hyperparathyroidism.
- Plasma parathyroid hormone is about three times the upper level of normal.
- Plasma renin and aldosterone are normal.
- Plasma 1,25-dihydroxycholecalciferol is low.
- Renal investigations show bilateral small scarred kidneys, due to reflux nephropathy.
- Maximum urine concentrating ability is 400 mosmol/l.

A 24-hour urine collection shows excretion of:
- 210 mmol sodium/day
- 75 mmol potassium/day
- 12 mmol creatinine/day when plasma creatinine is 0.25 mmol/l
- 420 μmol microalbumin/day.

Q14 Details of renal function such as GFR, renal blood flow, filtration fraction, etc. can be calculated from clearance formulae. Which one of the following formulae is *not* correct?

A. GFR = $\dfrac{\text{Urine flow rate} \times \text{Urine creatinine concentration}}{\text{Plasma creatinine concentration}}$

B. Filtration fraction = $\dfrac{\text{GFR}}{\text{Renal plasma flow}}$

C. Fractional excretion of x = $\dfrac{\text{Urine flow rate} \times \text{Urine concentration of } x}{\text{GFR} \times \text{Plasma concentration of } x}$

D. Free water clearance = Urine flow rate $- \left(\dfrac{\text{Urine osmolality} \times \text{Urine flow rate}}{\text{Plasma osmolality}} \right)$

E. Renal plasma flow = $\dfrac{\text{Renal blood flow} \times 100}{100 - \text{Haematocrit}\%}$

Q15 J.N.'s plasma creatinine is 0.25 mmol/l and his urine creatinine secretion is 12 mmol/day. What is his GFR?

A. 48 ml/min
B. 33 ml/min
C. 66 ml/min
D. 21 ml/min
E. 24 ml/min

Q16 Which of the following strategies would be of *least* importance in management of this patient?

A. treatment of blood pressure
B. restriction of dietary sodium
C. restriction of dietary protein
D. restriction of dietary phosphate
E. restriction of dietary potassium

Q17 In J.N. and other patients with chronic renal failure, which of the following is most likely *not* to be correct?

A. individual nephron GFR is elevated
B. individual nephron proximal tubule sodium absorption is increased
C. fractional absorption of sodium in the proximal tubule is decreased
D. the driving force for potassium secretion in the distal nephron is decreased
E. fractional absorption of sodium by the kidney is decreased

Q18 J.N.'s normochromic normocytic anaemia is most likely to be due to:

A. poor iron absorption
B. poor protein metabolism
C. low erythropoietin levels
D. increased red cell destruction
E. none of the above

J.N. is placed on a diet containing reduced protein (60 g/day) and reduced phosphate (difficult to achieve), and a restricted sodium intake of 70 mmol/day.

Two months later, his blood pressure is 155/90 mmHg and his plasma biochemistry is as follows:

Sodium	139 mmol/l
Potassium	4.6 mmol/l
Chloride	105 mmol/l
Bicarbonate	22 mmol/l
Calcium	2.32 mmol/l
Phosphate	1.78 mmol/l
Urea	12.4 mmol/l
Creatinine	0.23 mmol/l
pH	7.32

Q19 Which of the following procedures would be the preferable way to reduce the likelihood of progressive bone disease in this patient?

A. aluminium hydroxide orally
B. calcium carbonate orally
C. vitamin D orally
D. parathyroid hormone injections
E. calcitonin injections

This treatment results in a fall in plasma phosphate to 1.42 mmol/l and a rise in ionized calcium to 2.41 mmol/l.

An angiotensin-converting enzyme (ACE) inhibitor is added to his therapy and his blood pressure falls to 145/85 mmHg. However, since this value is still high for a young individual it is decided that his blood pressure needs better control and that a diuretic should be added.

Q20 Which of the following types of diuretic is most likely to be useful in this patient?

A. carbonic anhydrase inhibitors (e.g. acetazolamide)
B. loop diuretics (e.g. furosemide)
C. thiazide-type diuretics (e.g. hydrochlorothiazide)
D. sodium-channel inhibitors (e.g. amiloride)
E. aldosterone antagonists (e.g. spironolactone)

The appropriate diuretic is added to his therapy and his blood pressure falls to 132/74 mmHg. Good control of blood pressure is confirmed with a 24-hour ambulatory blood pressure measurement.

J.N. adheres to his diet and medications and stays well but over the next 3 years his renal function continues to deteriorate and his haemoglobin falls to 8.0 g/dl. He starts to tire more easily and is unable to do as much activity as before.

Erythropoietin is given and this improves his symptoms and raises his haemoglobin. However he continues to deteriorate. His plasma biochemistry 6 years after his presentation is:

Sodium	135 mmol/l
Potassium	5.1 mmol/l
Chloride	109 mmol/l
Bicarbonate	12 mmol/l
Calcium	1.88 mmol/l
Phosphate	2.02 mmol/l
Urea	25.4 mmol/l
Creatinine	0.62 mmol/l
pH	7.28

Twenty-four hour urine data are:

Volume	1.2 litres
Sodium	50 mmol/l
Potassium	40 mmol/l
Creatinine	9.3 mmol/l

Q21 His GFR as measured by creatinine clearance would now be:

A. 18 ml/min
B. 15 ml/min
C. 12.5 ml/min
D. 10 ml/min
E. 2 ml/min

Q22 At this time his body electrolyte content would most likely show:

A. total body potassium elevated
B. total body potassium reduced
C. total body sodium elevated
D. total body sodium reduced
E. no alteration in total body sodium or potassium

Q23 Which of the following would you administer to help correct his acidosis?

A. carbonic anhydrase inhibitors
B. sodium chloride
C. furosemide
D. sodium bicarbonate
E. potassium bicarbonate

Q24 Which of the following measures would be most indicated at this time to help improve his calcium metabolism?

A. parathyroidectomy
B. oral aluminium hydroxide
C. increased calcium carbonate administration
D. 1,25-dihydroxycholecalciferol
E. calcitonin injections

It is decided to place J.N. on dialysis with a view to transplantation. He is dialysed for six months and receives a kidney which is a compatible match from his mother.

The result is very successful. It is now 10 years post transplantation and his renal function is normal.

MCQ ANSWERS AND FEEDBACK

1.D. There is no evidence of nephrotic syndrome or glomerulonephritis (no protein and/or red cells in the urine). Renal artery stenosis rarely presents in the young as chronic renal failure. Polycystic kidneys can present with renal failure, but usually at an older age and there are no masses in the loins. The most likely cause is reflux nephropathy.

2.E. All of these are likely to be due to chronic renal failure with sodium retention leading to high blood pressure, absence of erythropoietin leading to anaemia and disturbance of calcium metabolism leading to bone disease.

3.A. With a plasma creatinine of 0.25 mmol/l both the plasma potassium and plasma calcium are likely to be normal. There will be a trend towards acidosis (low pH), but this will usually be in the normal range due to respiratory compensation. Most likely only bicarbonate will be low, due to impaired ability to excrete H^+. The other possibility (not listed) is that all values will be in the normal range.

4.C. Mechanistically, the retention of phosphate by the kidney is the trigger leading to bone disease. This reduces ionized calcium, which causes parathyroid hormone release. The two plasma values that are abnormal would be high phosphate and a high parathyroid hormone.

5.C. Parathyroid hormone and phosphate would be elevated (see Question 4). There is a defect in forming active vitamin D by the kidney. However, vitamin D itself would be normal and the addition of 25-hydroxyl by the liver is normal. The defect is that the 1-hydroxyl group cannot be added by the kidney.

6.E. High parathyroid hormone (see answers to Questions 3, 4 and 5).

7.B. All of these can cause secondary hypertension. The most common cause is an adrenal adenoma. Chronic renal disease with retention of sodium is the most common cause of secondary hypertension.

8.E. A renal secreting tumour will cause high plasma renin and high plasma angiotensin II, leading to high plasma aldosterone. This will cause sodium retention, loss of potassium (hypokalaemia) and severe hypertension. It is very uncommon. A renal artery stenosis also has most of these features, but the plasma renin may be normal in many situations.

9.B. Secretion of aldosterone by an adrenal adenoma causes sodium retention, hypokalaemia and moderate hypertension. The renin level is low (as is plasma angiotensin II) due to feedback from the sodium retention and the elevated blood pressure. Bilateral adrenal hyperplasia could produce a similar picture.

10.D. Episodic release of catecholamines by a phaeochromocytoma leads to severe episodic elevation of blood pressure. The plasma potassium is usually normal and plasma renin would be normal or possibly low if there is chronic blood pressure elevation.

11.A. Secretion of glucocorticosteroids by the adrenals due to the pituitary hypersecretion of adrenocorticotrophic hormone (ACTH) leads to Cushing's disease, which has these features.

12.A. The cause of this person's modest blood pressure elevation is probably retention of sodium. Mechanistically this leads to increased blood volume, increased cardiac output and increased blood pressure. However, chronically the pressure stays elevated due to increased peripheral resistance. Most likely plasma renin, plasma angiotensin II and aldosterone would be in the normal range or lower than normal.

13.A. Early in renal disease when GFR is still close to normal, the first defect is in maximum concentrating ability, reflecting a decreased number of functional nephrons. The normal

human kidney can concentrate up to 1200 mosmoles. All the other values are usually normal until GFR is <60 ml/min (see also Questions 3 and 4).

14.E. Plasma flow is less than blood flow, so the formula should be:

$$\text{Renal plasma flow} = \frac{\text{Renal blood flow} (100 - \text{Haematocrit})}{100}$$

15.B. $\text{GFR} = \dfrac{\text{Urine flow rate} \times \text{Urine creatinine concentration}}{\text{Plasma creatinine concentration}}$

or $\dfrac{\text{Timed creatinine excretion}}{\text{Plasma creatinine concentration}}$

$= \dfrac{12 \text{ mmol/day}}{0.25 \text{ mmol/l}} = 48 \text{ l/day} = \dfrac{48 \times 1000}{24 \times 60} \text{ ml/min}$

$= 33.3 \text{ ml/min}$

16.E. A protein-restricted diet (not severe, about 40 g/day) will reduce the acid load to be excreted; a sodium-restricted diet (around 70 mmol/day) may reduce blood pressure and if this is not normalized drug treatment will be needed. A phosphate-restricted diet (difficult to achieve) would reduce the phosphate load and thus interrupt the sequence leading to bone disease. Potassium restriction is usually not needed as, provided the urine output is greater than 1 litre/day, plasma potassium usually stays in the normal range. Excess potassium intake, for example dried fruits, should be avoided.

17.D. As renal failure takes place, the GFR of the remaining nephrons increases. This means more total sodium is reabsorbed by each proximal tubule, but the fractional reabsorption of sodium becomes less by both the proximal tubule and the kidney. There will be more sulphate in the distal nephron, leading to a greater driving force for potassium secretion and excretion.

18.C. Low erythropoietin levels are the most likely cause. In more severe renal disease, other factors also become important.

19.B. Oral calcium carbonate would be the preferred option. This combines with phosphate in the diet, reducing the amount absorbed and thereby reducing plasma phosphate. The extra calcium also allows more calcium to be absorbed, which also helps to reduce the progression of bone disease. Aluminium hydroxide also combines with phosphate in the diet and does reduce phosphate, but without the added advantage of extra calcium absorption. There is no indication for parathyroid hormone or calcitonin and oral vitamin D would be ineffective. J.N. was given 1200 mg $CaCO_3$/day, orally.

20.B. In a person with renal failure, the loop diuretics are the preferred drugs. Carbonic anhydrase inhibitors have little effect as bicarbonate is already low and thiazide diuretics are relatively ineffective. The potassium-sparing diuretics (amiloride and spironolactone) are usually contraindicated as they may cause H$^+$ and potassium retention.

21.C. $\text{GFR} = \dfrac{\text{Urine flow rate} \times \text{Urine creatinine concentration}}{\text{Plasma creatinine concentration}}$

or $\dfrac{\text{Timed creatinine excretion}}{\text{Plasma creatinine concentration}}$

$= \dfrac{1.2 \times 9.3}{0.62}$ litres/day = 18 litres/day

$= \dfrac{8 \times 1000}{24 \times 60}$ ml/min = 12.5 ml/min

22.B. Total body sodium is probably normal as blood pressure is normal, there is no oedema and plasma sodium is in the normal range. Plasma potassium is elevated, but the extracellular fluid represents only a small fraction of total body potassium (normally about 50 mmol of a total 2000 mmol).

However, acidosis (pH = 7.28) causes potassium to come out of cells and this potassium is lost in the urine, so total body potassium is almost certainly reduced.

23.D. Carbonic anhydrase inhibitors would have little effect, and by causing loss of bicarbonate, could make the acidosis worse. Sodium chloride and furosemide would have little effect on acidosis. Potassium bicarbonate and sodium bicarbonate would both correct the acidosis, but as plasma potassium is elevated, it would be preferable to use sodium bicarbonate initially.

24.D. At this time, the bone disease is progressive with a low plasma calcium. It would probably be preferable to give 1,25-dihydroxycholecalciferol to improve calcium absorption. The phosphate is elevated but not excessive, so it is not necessary to reduce phosphate absorption. Occasionally the parathyroid glands can become autonomous and a parathyroidectomy may be needed but, when this happens, plasma calcium is usually elevated. The implementation of dialysis should correct plasma phosphate and, by increasing calcium absorption with active vitamin D, progressive bone disease will hopefully be prevented.

CASE REVIEW

Unexplained renal failure in an adolescent can be due to a number of causes. Polycystic kidneys are inherited and may present at this age or (more commonly) later with chronic failure, but there was no family history and the kidneys were not palpable. Glomerular damage as a result of immune disease could be the cause but there would usually be blood and/or protein in the urine. Nephrotic syndrome is usually associated with glomerular damage and always with proteinuria. Vascular disease is a cause of renal failure in older people and acute vasculitis can occur in young people but would usually have associated haematuria and would occur only acutely.

The most likely cause is reflux nephropathy in which in young children there is reflux from the bladder into the kidneys on one or both sides. This causes damage and scarring and the kidney does not grow adequately. There is often little problem until puberty when there are increased demands on the kidney and the functional reserve is exceeded. To cause problems the disease must be bilateral because the kidneys have a large reserve of function. When a kidney is removed or is diseased the remaining nephrons increase their GFR, so that there is a much smaller reduction in overall GFR than might be predicted. Even if one kidney is completely removed, GFR falls only from 120 to 100 ml/min.

In most situations, as renal impairment starts the first function to deteriorate is the urinary concentrating ability. Serum creatinine stays in the normal range until GFR is only about 50–60% of normal, which corresponds to about 60–70% of nephrons having been destroyed. In chronic renal disease plasma sodium is usually normal and, provided the urine volume is greater than 1 litre/day, plasma potassium is usually in the normal range.

One of the first plasma variables to rise is plasma phosphate because its excretion is highly dependent on GFR. It is filtered at the glomerulus and reabsorbed in the proximal tubule in direct proportion to sodium and water. When plasma phosphate becomes elevated this combines with calcium to reduce the ionized calcium level, leading to increased parathyroid hormone secretion. This acts on bone to release calcium and phosphate and also on the kidney to suppress proximal tubular reabsorption of sodium and water. This means less calcium and phosphate are absorbed in the proximal tubule. The excretion of phosphate is consequently increased because it is not absorbed to any major extent in the rest of the nephron. However, parathyroid hormone stimulates the absorption of calcium by the loop of Henle and the distal nephron. Thus, in early renal failure, plasma phosphate is mildly elevated, parathyroid hormone is elevated but plasma calcium is usually in the normal range. The maintained elevated parathyroid hormone levels will eventually lead to bone disease (*hyperparathyroidism*) (Fig. 16.1). This can be prevented at least in part by reducing intestinal phosphate absorption and keeping plasma phosphate normal.

Parathyroid hormone is also important in the formation of active vitamin D (1,25-dihydroxycholecalciferol). The attachment of the 1-hydroxy group by the kidney cells is the rate-limiting step and this step is stimulated by parathyroid hormone. Vitamin D increases calcium absorption from the bowel and also is important in its deposition into bone. To assist in the calcium and phosphate bone problems associated with excess parathyroid hormone, calcium carbonate can be given orally. This combines with phosphate in the diet to form insoluble calcium phosphate complexes in the intestine, which are not absorbed. The additional calcium also increases total calcium absorption. When the plasma calcium level falls and bone disease is progressive, vitamin D administration may be needed. However, it needs to be in the form of the active vitamin (1,25-dihydroxycholecalciferol).

Impaired kidney function reduces the capacity to conserve and/or excrete various ions including sodium, potassium and protons. Plasma sodium usually stays in the normal range but if there is excessive sodium intake the kidney's excretory capacity is exceeded and blood pressure rises to restore balance. By contrast, if sodium intake is reduced too much the kidney is unable to conserve sodium and the person may be volume-depleted and hypotensive. Potassium levels are usually in the normal range provided urine volume is greater than 1 litre/day because the retention of SO_4^{2-} and its excretion in the urine cause a higher potential difference in the collecting system, allowing K^+ secretion to be increased and thus excretion is maintained. Secretion and excretion of H^+ is impaired and there is retention in the body. This does not result in a major change in pH because of respiratory compensations. However, plasma bicarbonate will fall and $Paco_2$ will also fall. When the pH falls this will cause a shift in potassium equilibrium between cells and plasma and more potassium will come out of the cells, causing plasma potassium to rise. This will cause a greater loss of potassium in the urine and thus although plasma potassium may be elevated, total body potassium may be reduced. If the pH falls, sodium bicarbonate can be given.

The retention of sodium will usually cause blood pressure to rise. It is important to reverse this because hypertension increases the rate of progression of renal disease. Some common causes of hypertension are listed in Table 16.1.

ACE inhibitors and the angiotensin type 1-receptor blocking drugs appear to prevent the progression of renal failure better than other drugs, though there is often initially a rise in

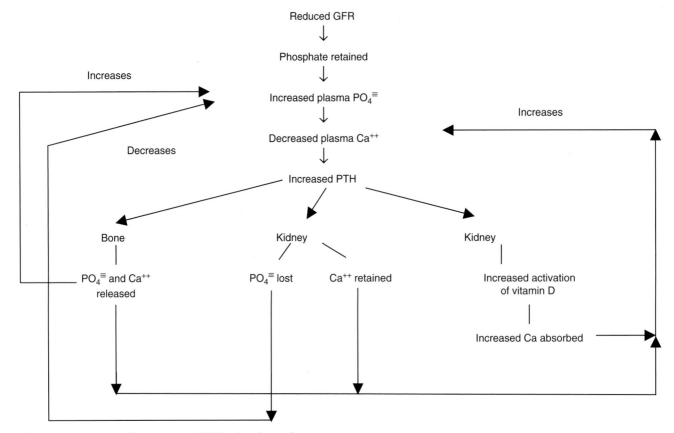

Fig. 16.1 Mechanism of how reduced GFR leads to bone disease.

Table 16.1 Common causes of hypertension. Note that most types of hypertension involve sodium retention

Types of hypertension	Causal factors
Primary (essential) hypertension	Diet and lifestyle (high Na$^+$, low K$^+$, obesity, lack of exercise)
Secondary hypertension	
Renal impairment	Sodium retention
Renal artery stenosis	Renin secretion
Adrenal adenoma	Aldosterone secretion
Adrenal hyperplasia	Glucocorticoid hypersecretion
Phaeochromocytoma	Excess catecholamine secretion

creatinine and a fall in GFR. To allow a full effect the patient should have a reduced sodium intake and, if that is not sufficient, a diuretic should be added. A loop diuretic is usually used (furosemide) because thiazides are relatively ineffective in renal failure and the potassium-sparing diuretics (aldosterone antagonists and amiloride) are usually contraindicated due to the hyperkalaemia.

The kidney produces erythropoietin, which is important for normal red cell formation. As renal failure progresses, production of this hormone is impaired and anaemia of the normochromic normocytic type results. Renal failure may have no symptoms until GFR <30% of normal. In chronic renal failure metabolic problems predominate:

- No erythropoietin → anaemia
- No activation of vitamin D → bone disease
- Sodium retention → increased blood pressure
- Phosphate retained → low ionized calcium → raised parathyroid hormone → bone disease.

Poor protein metabolism may also contribute to the anaemia.

Treatment of the underlying process is usually not successful in reversing chronic renal failure, so effective treatment consists of measures to prevent its progression. One of these, as discussed above, is treatment of elevated blood pressure, with reduced NaCl diet and/or drugs. Second, dietary interventions can be used, with reduced protein intake reducing the H$^+$ load and reduced phosphate absorption preventing bone disease. When dietary control fails to prevent problems dialysis may be needed (haemodialysis, peritoneal dialysis) and, in appropriate cases, transplantation.

As renal failure becomes more severe specific additional measures may be needed.

- Bone disease – active vitamin D; parathyroidectomy
- Anaemia – erythropoietin
- Hypertension – drugs and sodium balance
- Acidosis – sodium bicarbonate.

A person with severe renal disease may be maintained alive but it is important to initiate dialysis before irreversible or difficult to reverse changes are established.

KEY POINTS

- Renal failure is frequently silent and signs and symptoms may not occur until GFR is 30% of normal.
- Signs and symptoms of chronic renal failure are due to metabolic consequences.
- Anaemia, bone disease and hypertension are common presentations.
- Anaemia is due to lack of erythropoietin.
- Early bone disease is due to phosphate retention leading to hyperparathyroidism.
- Bone disease is also due to inadequate amount of renal tissue to form active vitamin D.
- Hypertension is due to Na$^+$ retention.

ADDITIONAL READING

Braunwald E *et al.* (2001) *Harrison's Principles of Internal Medicine*, 15th edition. McGraw-Hill, New York.

Seldin DW & Giebisch G (2000) *The Kidney: Physiology and Pathophysiology*, 3rd edition. Lippincott Williams & Wilkins, Philadelphia.

Souhami RL & Moxham T (2002) *Textbook of Medicine*, 4th edition. Churchill Livingstone, London.

Whitworth JA & Lawrence JR (1994) *Textbook of Renal Disease*, 2nd edition. Churchill Livingstone, Edinburgh.

A marathon in the tropics

CASE AND MCQS

Case introduction

A half-marathon road race is being organized in Kuala Lumpur in aid of charity. As a trainee in cardiac rehabilitation, you have been asked to act as medical officer for the event. You will be responsible for checking the entrants' fitness to take part, advising on the health and safety aspects of the race and ensuring that adequate medical cover is provided during the event.

One of your first tasks when people begin to put their names down as entrants is to screen them for contraindications to endurance exercise and to assess their absolute fitness, so you can advise them on the appropriate race time for which they should be aiming.

Q1 Absolute physical fitness can be quantified by measurement of:

A. plasma lactate level during maximal exercise
B. oxygen consumption during maximal exercise
C. carbon dioxide production during maximal exercise
D. oxygen consumption at a given submaximal workload
E. either B or D

Q2 A typical value for $V_{O_{2max}}$ in a young, healthy sedentary man would be around:

A. 3 (ml/min)/kg
B. 5 (ml/min)/kg
C. 30 (ml/min)/kg
D. 50 (ml/min)/kg
E. 70 (ml/min)/kg

Q3 In women, $V_{O_{2max}}$ per unit body mass is around 20% lower than in men of the same age. What factors can you think of that would explain this dramatic difference in work capacity?

Although determination of $V_{O_{2max}}$ is the accepted standard for quantifying work capacity, frequent repetition of this test is time-consuming and sometimes inconvenient. If you are concerned to monitor an individual's fitness over time, this can be tracked reasonably accurately by measuring heart rate rises in response to a given level of work.

Q4 The maximal heart rate that can be achieved during exercise:

A. never exceeds 200 beats/min
B. can be approximated as (200 – age in years) beats/min
C. is higher in obese than in lean individuals
D. is higher at age 20 years than at age 50 years
E. is higher in young adults than in children

Q5 At sea level, the workload that can be accomplished during acute exercise is limited primarily by:

A. lung volume
B. respiratory muscle efficiency
C. alveolar oxygen diffusion
D. cardiac emptying time
E. cardiac filling time

Q6 Physical training, such as a rehabilitation programme, improves exercise capacity by affecting a number of cardiovascular parameters. Which of the following parameters is *not* increased during training?

A. stroke volume
B. cardiac filling time
C. haematocrit
D. skeletal muscle capillary density
E. blood volume

With the approach of race day, you have to give sensible advice to the participants on how to tailor their nutrient and fluid intakes before and during the race, in order to optimize energy output and maintain water and electrolyte balance. At this time, it is worth spending a few minutes revizing the regulation of energy substrate availability and of fluid balance.

Let us start by thinking about food ingestion and the possible impact on energy substrates. What would be the best sort of pre-event meal for an endurance athlete?

Q7 Would you recommend:

A. a high-protein meal 3–4 hours before the event
B. a high-carbohydrate meal 3–4 hours before the event
C. a high-carbohydrate meal 1–2 hours before the event
D. a high-protein meal 1–2 hours before the event
E. a balanced meal no less than 12 hours before the event

Next, consider whether it would be beneficial to ingest energy substrates during the race itself.

Q8 The best strategy for food ingestion during endurance exercise is:

A. no food because digestion will divert blood from exercising muscles
B. no food because it will cause insulin secretion and inhibit glycogenolysis
C. glucose tablets because this will help maintain blood glucose
D. energy bars because the protein content will enhance glucose absorption
E. fructose because this is absorbed more rapidly than glucose

Now we should consider how to maintain fluid balance during the race. This will involve considering sweat production and also any fluid redistribution that might occur within the body. Any difficulties in maintaining adequate fluid balance will be exacerbated in a climate such as Kuala Lumpur's, where environmental temperature and humidity are both extremely high.

As a beginning, let us think about fluid distribution. During sustained exercise, plasma volume falls rapidly over the first few minutes and then continues to decline much more slowly. Look at the magnitude and time course of these changes (Fig. 17.1) and think about the underlying reasons.

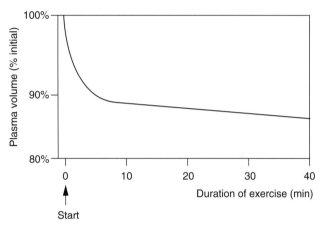

Fig. 17.1 Effect of 40 minutes sustained whole-body exercise on plasma volume.

Q9 The fall in circulating plasma volume during the first few minutes of whole-body aerobic exercise is caused by:

A. extravasation due to vasodilation in exercising muscles
B. extravasation due to vasodilation in skin
C. trapping of blood in vasoconstricted splanchnic and renal beds
D. trapping of blood in pulmonary veins due to decreased intrathoracic pressure
E. sweat secretion due to rapid build-up of metabolic heat

Now let us consider the composition and volume of sweat that is normally produced and how these are changed by exercise and thermal stress. Remember that eccrine sweat is basically an ultrafiltrate of plasma, but that its composition is usually modified in the sweat ducts. Table 17.1 lists of values for whole-body eccrine sweating characteristic of people in certain environments.

Table 17.1 Volumes and sodium concentrations of sweat: options for Questions 10–12

	Volume of sweat (ml/h)	Sodium concentration of sweat (mmol/l)
A.	20	5
B.	20	140
C.	1000	50
D.	1000	5
E.	2000	50
F.	2000	5
G.	2000	140
H.	4000	5

Q10 Which of the options in Table 17.1 is characteristic of an individual who is acclimatized to a cool environment and who is at rest in the shade?

Q11 Which of the options in Table 17.1 is characteristic of an individual who is acclimatized to a cool environment and who is exercising heavily?

Q12 Which of the options in Table 17.1 is characteristic of an individual who is acclimatized to a hot environment and who is exercising heavily?

Q13 An individual is sweating at a rate of 1000 ml/h and the sweat contains 50 mmol/l sodium. Approximately how much salt (sodium chloride, MW = 58) would have to be ingested in order to maintain sodium balance?

A. around 100 mg/h
B. around 1 g/h
C. around 2.5 g/h
D. around 10 g/h
E. around 25 g/h

If an individual who is losing large amounts of sodium and water by sweating replaces the water but not the sodium, hyponatraemia will result. When plasma sodium falls to less than 125 mmol/l, neuronal and muscular functions are disturbed, leading to muscle cramps, nausea and lethargy.

Think about the roles of sodium in cellular homeostasis and decide the most likely mechanism by which these effects of hyponatraemia on nerve and muscle function are most likely to occur.

Q14 A reduction in extracellular fluid (ECF) sodium from 145 mmol/l to 120 mmol/l is likely to affect cell excitability because:

A. the fall in ECF osmolality causes cellular oedema
B. the fall in ECF osmolality causes cellular dehydration
C. the fall in ECF sodium reduces action potential amplitude
D. the fall in ECF sodium depolarizes the cells
E. the fall in ECF sodium hyperpolarizes the cells

As well as deciding on the absolute quantities of water and salt that might be needed for fluid balance, the rates of gastric emptying and intestinal absorption must be considered. No matter how much fluid is drunk, there is a limit to the rate at which fluid leaves the stomach. This is around 1200 ml/h at rest and, because of reduced gastric motility, only around 800 ml/h during exercise. For reasons of comfort, it is better for this volume to be drunk in relatively small amounts rather than all at once. The temperature of the fluid does not seem to affect emptying rate, although cool liquid is preferable from the viewpoint of temperature regulation. On the other hand, very cold liquid is difficult to drink quickly.

Gastric emptying rates are virtually identical for water or water containing electrolytes, but the solutes can affect intestinal absorption. Think about the processes involved with movement of substances across the intestinal epithelium and decide how to provide the most efficient absorption of water and sodium.

Q15 Maintenance of water and electrolyte balance would be most efficiently achieved by ingestion of which of the following?

A. water plus salt tablets
B. hypotonic saline
C. isotonic saline
D. hypertonic saline
E. any of A–D are equally effective

Q16 Fluid absorption could be enhanced further by inclusion of a small amount of glucose in the ingested solution. This is because glucose in the intestinal lumen:

A. increases the intraluminal/intracellular sodium gradient
B. stimulates pancreatic amylase secretion
C. activates epithelial water channels
D. provides energy for epithelial uptake pumps
E. stimulates sodium uptake

So now you have screened all the participants and have planned optimal advice on dietary preparation and for maintaining fluid balance. Even with these precautions, however, it is likely that a small number of participants may collapse during the race. We therefore need to think about the possible causes of collapse and how the disordered physiology of these patients can be restored to normal.

Q17 Collapse during endurance exercise in a hot, humid climate is most likely to be caused by:

A. reduced cerebral perfusion due to reduced plasma volume
B. reduced muscle perfusion due to reduced plasma volume
C. depletion of energy substrates
D. increased core temperature due to failure of sweating
E. increased core temperature due to reduced skin perfusion

Q18 In an individual who has collapsed in this way, what is the most urgent aspect of treatment?

A. restoration of normal brain blood flow
B. restoration of normal extracellular sodium concentration
C. restoration of normal plasma volume
D. removal of body heat
E. provision of glucose for cerebral metabolism

Q19 Removal of body heat under these circumstances could be achieved most effectively by:

A. ingestion of ice-cold water
B. blowing a fan on the skin
C. sponging the skin with an ice-pack
D. sponging the skin with tap water
E. immersing the individual in luke-warm water

MCQ ANSWERS AND FEEDBACK

1.B. The maximal rate of oxygen consumption during acute exercise (Vo_{2max} or Vo_{2peak}) is the standard parameter for quantifying fitness level. Although a person's capacity to produce work rises with their fitness, a given submaximal workload is associated with the same amount of oxygen consumption regardless of fitness, because the amount of muscle work remains constant. Increased fitness is associated with more lactate and carbon dioxide production at maximal workload but, since these markers reflect a mixture of aerobic and anaerobic metabolic pathways, they do not provide as linear an index of fitness as oxygen usage.

2.D. Typically, oxygen consumption rises 15-fold above resting levels during maximal exercise in an untrained individual. A 70-kg person consumes around 250 ml/min of oxygen at rest, so maximum consumption is therefore around (250×15) ml/min, which equates to about 50 (ml/min)/kg. The value of 30 (ml/min)/kg would be appropriate for an eld-

erly person, because ageing is associated with reduced muscle bulk and cardiac reserve. The figure of 70 (ml/min)/kg would be expected in a highly trained athlete, primarily because cardiovascular adaptations increase the efficiency of oxygen delivery to the muscles.

3. There are three reasons. Women have smaller hearts relative to their body mass than do men, so they have less capacity to increase cardiac output and muscle perfusion. As well, men have higher haematocrits because of the erythropoietic effect of testosterone. Finally, testosterone and oestrogens have differential actions on deposition of muscle and fat cells, so that women have a lower proportional contribution of muscle tissue to body mass.

4.D. The maximum frequency at which the sino-atrial node can generate action potentials is around 220 beats/min. This falls progressively with age, so at any age the maximal rate achievable is approximated by the calculation (220 − age in years) beats/min. In obese individuals (BMI >30 kg/m²), maximal rates are more accurately calculated by (200 − 1/2 age in years) beats/min. These formulae are reasonably accurate but there is in practice some variability between people. For each individual it is therefore useful to check the calculated value against that measured during a real Vo_{2max} test on at least one occasion.

5.E. In order for the ventricles to eject blood effectively, they must remain contracted for several hundred milliseconds. The sustained contraction is achieved by the long opening time of the voltage-gated calcium channels that produces the plateau of the ventricular action potential and sustained diffusion of extracellular calcium ions into the sarcomeres. At resting heart rates, this period lasts around 300 ms. In the presence of noradrenaline (norepinephrine) released from sympathetic nerves, calcium channel opening is shortened, with the action potential plateau and ventricular contraction lasting as little as 200 ms. This is essential for ventricular relaxation and filling to be maintained. Nonetheless, at near-maximal rates the absolute volume of blood that can enter the ventricles is severely limited by the very short diastolic period. You can see from Fig. 17.2 how the slow filling phase of diastole virtually disappears at 180 beats/min, while it is substantial at 60 beats/min.

At sea level, none of the processes involved in respiratory provision of oxygen impose any limitation on exercise capacity.

6.C. Repetitive exercise elevates blood volume by up to around 15%. This involves an initial retention of water due to potassium-induced aldosterone secretion, with subsequent stimulation of plasma protein synthesis by cortisol and of erythropoiesis by erythropoietin. However, this sequence of processes does not result in any net increase in haematocrit. Training also induces eccentric ventricular hypertrophy, with increased chamber volume and therefore increased stroke volume. As resting oxygen demand and cardiac output are unaltered, there is a compensatory fall in resting heart rate, which means more time is available for cardiac filling at all submaximal levels of cardiac output. A further response to training is growth of new capillaries in the exercised muscles, apparently as a result of local growth factor release from the muscle cells.

7.B. Optimal provision of metabolic energy relies on maximal glycogen availability. The liver represents the main store of glycogen and this is depleted progressively by ongoing metabolism even at rest, so by 12 hours after a meal, metabolic efficiency is far from optimal. Over shorter time intervals, the relative effectiveness of protein and carbohydrate as energy sources must be taken into account. Per unit oxygen con-sumed, protein generates only two-thirds as much energy as carbohydrate. In addition, protein remains in the stomach longer because it inhibits gastric motility. Carbohydrate feeding is therefore much more efficient as a source of glycogenesis.

Eating 3–4 hours before exercise allows sufficient time for all the glucose to be stored and for plasma insulin to restabilize. If the meal is only 1–2 hours before exercise, circulating glucose and insulin may still be elevated when exercise begins. Because insulin inhibits both gluconeogenesis and hepatic glycogenolysis, this may result in suboptimal glucose availability early in the exercise period.

8.C. Small amounts (about 25 g/h) of carbohydrate ingested at 15- to 30-minute intervals during endurance exercise delay depletion of glycogen stores and the consequent onset of fatigue. Glucose and fructose are absorbed at similar rates, but fructose is not as useful because it may cause abdominal discomfort. As long as the volume ingested is small, only an insignificant diversion of blood flow to the gastrointestinal tract occurs. Energy bars are less effective than glucose itself because they contain protein and fat. These slow up gastric emptying and increase gastrointestinal secretory activity, so cause more diversion of blood flow from muscle. Although carbohydrate absorption usually causes insulin secretion and depresses glycogenolysis, this does not occur during exercise because the associated sympathetic nervous system activation inhibits insulin release and stimulates glycogen breakdown.

9.A. The onset of skeletal muscle contraction is accompanied by immediate arteriolar vasodilation, mediated by local metabolites. The reduction in precapillary resistance elevates capillary hydrostatic pressure to values of 50–60 mmHg, substantially higher than can be balanced by plasma oncotic pressure, so there is water movement into the interstitium. This lowers plasma volume by around 12% over the first 10 minutes of whole-body exercise, and so rapidly imposes a new limit on cardiac output.

At very high workloads, water movement out of the plasma is stimulated further by increased intracellular metabolite accumulation creating an osmotic gradient. With continued activity, the heat of muscle metabolism will lead to sweat secretion, but the volume of sweat produced over the initial few minutes of exercise is trivial.

10.A. As an ultrafiltrate of plasma, secreted sweat must have an electrolyte composition similar to that of plasma, so the sodium concentration must be of the order of 140 mmol/l. However, unless the secretion rate is high, most of this sodium is reabsorbed as the sweat passes along the ducts. Because the reabsorptive process is selective for sodium, the final fluid contains much higher concentrations of some other substances (in particular potassium, urea and lactic acid) than are in plasma.

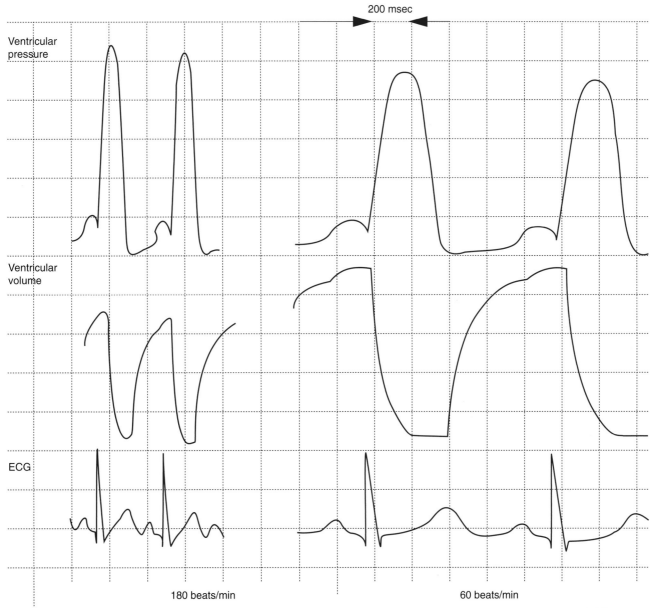

200 msec

Ventricular pressure

Ventricular volume

ECG

180 beats/min

60 beats/min

Fig. 17.2 Comparison of ventricular pressure and volume changes at heart rates of 180 and 60 beats/min. Note the marked difference in stroke volume.

11.C. Even with extreme heat stress, a person who is not ac-climatized to hot conditions is unable to produce sweat at greater volumes than around 1 litre/h. Production is limited by sodium reabsorption in the ducts, which reduces the intra-luminal osmolality and so causes osmotic water reabsorption. As the time available for reabsorption in the ducts is shorter at high secretion rates, the final sweat has a much higher sodium concentration than under thermoneutral conditions.

12.F. Acclimatization to hot conditions over periods of sev-eral weeks causes a dramatic increase in the volume of sweat that can be produced in response to heat stress. This is due to

glandular hypertrophy in response to increased activation. In addition, the sodium depletion caused by the initial sweat-ing response to heat increases aldosterone secretion. As in the kidney, sodium reabsorption in the sweat ducts is enhanced by aldosterone. At high secretory rates, the heat-acclimatized person therefore produces sweat with a much lower sodium concentration than occurs in unacclimatized individuals. This has the obvious biological advantage of conserving whole-body sodium stores.

13.C. Loss of 1000 ml fluid containing 50 mmol/l sodium means that a total of 50 mmol sodium has been lost. This represents approximately (50×23) mg or 1.15 g sodium, which is equivalent to about 2.5 g (half a teaspoon) of sodium chloride.

14.A. As sodium ions represent around half of the osmotically active particles in plasma and extracellular fluid, hyponatraemia will reduce total extracellular osmolality and extracellular water will diffuse down the osmotic gradient into cells. The cellular oedema that results interferes with cellular signalling pathways and alters membrane excitability by physical distortion. Because the cell membrane is virtually impermeable to sodium at rest, alterations in extracellular sodium do not affect the internal concentration of around 10 mmol/l, so there is still a high transmembrane concentration gradient to provide rapid sodium movement into cells when voltage-gated channels open during an action potential. Sodium impermeability of the cell membrane at rest also means that variations in extracellular concentration do not affect resting membrane potential.

In situations where hyponatraemia has developed rapidly, rapid restoration of normal sodium levels is important in order to avoid central nervous system damage. Where sodium depletion has developed chronically, on the other hand, compensatory adjustments of cellular osmolality have taken place. Under these circumstances, rapid replacement of normal plasma sodium would cause osmotic cell dehydration. This can also result in central nervous system damage.

15.B. Absorption of water from the small intestine is more efficient when the intraluminal contents are hypotonic, because this creates the best osmotic gradient. We decided in Question 12 that about 2.5 g salt is needed to replace the sodium lost with every litre of water. A solution of 2.5 g salt in 1 litre water (that is, 0.25% saline) is considerably hypotonic to extracellular fluid, which is equivalent to 0.9% saline. Ingestion of salt in solid form would be much less efficient than drinking saline, since the high local osmolality would limit absorption.

16.E. As in the proximal renal tubule, some sodium absorption across the luminal membrane of the jejunal epithelium is via sodium–proton countertransport, but some is by carriage on a co-transporter with glucose or amino acids. The presence of glucose in the jejunal lumen therefore increases uptake of sodium and of the water that follows it by osmotic attraction. Activation of this glucose–sodium co-transporter is the underlying principle of oral rehydration therapy in cases of infective diarrhoea. The bacterial toxins inhibit sodium–proton movement, so body fluid replenishment cannot be achieved by drinking water or saline alone. However, the glucose co-transporter is not affected by infection. Both water and sodium can therefore be absorbed effectively if small amounts of glucose are added to the ingested saline.

In practice, the absence of sodium and water uptake also leads to loss of potassium and bicarbonate, so rehydration fluid should contain these as well as sodium. One standard formula is 3/4 teaspoon table salt, 1 teaspoon baking soda, one cup orange juice (to supply potassium) and 4 tablespoons sugar, in 1 litre of water.

17.A. The thermal stress of exercising produces very rapid fluid depletion, especially in a humid environment that limits the evaporative efficiency of sweating. Almost all of this fluid will be drawn from the plasma. Without adequate fluid replacement, venous return and cardiac output will fall progressively and, because of the gravitational field involved, this will preferentially reduce cerebral perfusion pressure and cause fainting. If blood pressure falls, then cutaneous perfusion and sweat secretion will also be reduced, impairing heat loss and leading to hyperthermia. In an upright individual, however, the hypotensive fall in cerebral perfusion will cause collapse before hyperthermia occurs.

18.D. Once the gravitational stress of upright posture is removed, the pronounced autoregulatory capacity of the cerebral vascular bed will restore brain blood flow to a normal level. However, autoregulation is not present in the cutaneous vasculature, so skin blood flow and sweat production remain low. As a result, metabolic heat from the skeletal muscles causes core temperature to rise rapidly. As brain function is irreversibly damaged at temperatures above 41°C, rapid restoration of adequate heat loss processes is the essential aim in treating these patients.

19.D. The skin is the only pathway by which heat can be removed rapidly from the bloodstream. Although cold water in the stomach will cool blood passing through the gastric circulation, this makes only a small contribution to total venous return and in any case a collapsed patient is unlikely to be able to drink large volumes of cold fluid. Heat loss through the skin relies on creating a suitable thermal gradient, either by conduction, convection or evaporation. But the first two of these are effective only when there is a large temperature gradient between body and environment. Thus, immersion in cold water is effective, but luke-warm water creates too small a gradient for rapid cooling. Similarly, creating convective currents with a fan is useful only when the air temperature is very low or when evaporative cooling occurs in parallel because the skin has been wetted.

In theory, sponging the skin with ice would provide some local cooling as well as initiating evaporation but, in practice, it is better to use water that is not ice-cold. Very low temperatures stimulate cutaneous cold receptors and initiate reflex vasoconstriction in the skin, which limits heat removal from the deeper tissues.

CASE REVIEW

Exercise confers substantial protection against cardiovascular disease and plays a central role in therapy of and rehabilitation after a wide range of disorders. In addition, measurement of cardiopulmonary changes during standardized exercise protocols is an essential tool for assessing patients with cardiorespiratory disease. For all these reasons, it is important that a medical graduate understands something of exercise physiology and the principles of fitness evaluation.

In this chapter, the metabolic cost of exercise has been discussed in terms of millilitres of oxygen consumed per unit time and unit body mass, since that is a convenient way to compare basal and activity-induced oxygen usage. The unit of (ml/min)/kg is widely used in exercise physiology but, for clinical assessment of patients, it is more convenient to use the metabolic equivalent, or MET. One MET equals an oxygen usage of 3.5 (ml/min)/kg and so provides a comprehensive range of exercise capacities that can be expressed in terms of single figures (Table 17.2).

Several standard protocols exist for assessing exercise capacity. These involve progressively increased work intensities on an ergometer, reaching the subject's maximal capacity within a total period of around 10 minutes. Most protocols are based on step-wise increases in workload but, in some, the steps are too large to allow accurate evaluation of individuals with limited work capacity. The test of choice therefore depends on the population being studied and for a patient whose MET limit is around 5 it is preferable to use a protocol that provides ramped rather than stepped increases in workload.

The choice of ergometer also depends on the circumstances. Treadmill walking recruits a slightly higher proportion of whole-body musculature than does cycling, so the measured work capacity is greater. On the other hand, treadmills are larger and noisier than cycles, and unsuitable for patients who require physical support during exercise. As well, absolute workload can be quantified more precisely with the cycle, which is an important issue when assessing circulatory efficiency.

Table 17.2 Representative MET values used for classification of fitness and mobility levels

Oxygen usage ((ml/min)/kg)	METs	Classification
82.5	24	Olympic athlete
45.5	13	Typical normal young sedentary
35.5	10	Typical normal middle-aged sedentary
17.5	5	Minimal activity level for daily life

Absolute heart rates during graded exercise cannot be used to monitor changes in fitness, because resting heart rate falls during training. The important factor is the proportion of the available range of tachycardia that has to be used in order to provide cardiac output at the given workload – that is, the heart rate reserve. To determine this, the difference between resting and predicted maximum rates is calculated and the exercise-induced increment is expressed as a percentage of that difference.

When performing these calculations, it is important to remember that heart rates at rest during the day are often significantly elevated by central arousal and increased metabolic rate. The most valid measurement of true resting heart rate is one taken immediately after waking in the morning, while the subject is still supine. Of course, heart rate is of no value in assessing exercise capacity when the normal processes for producing sympathetic tachycardia are impaired; for instance in post-infarct patients treated with a beta-adrenoreceptor antagonist.

Overheating is a continual potential hazard during exercise. Even a moderate workload raises metabolic heat production four- to five-fold, to levels around 2000 kJ/h (approx. 500 kcal/h). If this heat remained inside the body, core temperature would rise by 4°C/h. The situation is compounded by the facts that raised temperature itself increases cellular metabolic rate and that the body fluids act as a large heat store. As a result, core temperature during sustained whole-body exercise is always somewhat above the value at rest. During endurance exercise such as a road race or cross-country running, values as high as 39.5°C are common.

So long as heat exchange processes are efficient, this moderate hyperthermia has no deleterious effect and can even facilitate heat loss by increasing the thermal gradient between skin and environment. Nonetheless, irreversible brain damage will occur if core temperature exceeds 41°C, so the safety margin is small. High air humidity, high air temperature and solar radiation will all reduce the efficiency of heat loss. In these circumstances, even short periods of plasma volume depletion to an level that reduces sweat secretion and skin blood flow can have disastrous consequences.

Because of the large amount of heat produced, by even resting metabolism, impairment of heat loss processes can lead to hyperthermia in a variety of susceptible patient groups. These include individuals who are fluid-depleted or have impaired capacity to increase their cardiac output and peripheral perfusion, obese individuals in whom the skin represents a much more efficient insulative layer than normal and those in whom there has been damage to the sweat ducts by burns or skin disease.

Effective treatment of overheating relies on recognizing whether the underlying problem is depletion of effective plasma volume (*heat exhaustion*) or true hyperthermia (*heat stroke*). But, as described above, the first problem can rapidly lead to the second under conditions where core temperature is already elevated. So, treatment of an individual who has collapsed during physical activity often needs to address fluid replacement and cooling at the same time.

For emergency purposes, evaporation is an effective process that does not rely on using cold fluid to bath the skin. If available, however, ice packs applied to regions where large veins travel close to the surface – neck, armpit and groin – speed up the process. Application of very cold objects to wider areas of skin should be avoided because it causes reflex cutaneous vasoconstriction. If there is access to running water, placing the patient under a cool (but not cold) shower offers the joint benefits of evaporative and conductive heat loss.

KEY POINTS

- Assessment of work capacity is an important aspect of clinical diagnosis and therapy.
- Standard protocols for assessing work capacity, or fitness, are well established but the choice of protocol depends on the patient group being evaluated.
- Exercise capacity is normally limited at sea level by the finite capacity of the heart to pump adequate blood.
- As exercise continues, further limits at any work intensity are imposed by plasma extravasation, by competition between muscle and skin perfusion and by progressive fluid depletion due to sweating.

- Optimal energy and fluid replacement during exercise requires detailed consideration of digestive tract physiology.
- Unless adequate fluid replacement occurs, plasma volume falls rapidly during sustained exercise, with failure of the normal pathways for heat loss and a rapid rise in core temperature.
- If this occurs, reduction of body temperature must be achieved as a matter of urgency in order to prevent irreversible brain damage.
- During the cooling process, a central issue is to avoid reflex vasoconstriction in the skin that would hinder heat loss.

ADDITIONAL READING

Bell C & O'Sullivan SE (2005) Cardiovascular responses to exercise. In *Exercise in the Prevention and Treatment of Disease*, J Gormley & J. Hussey (eds). Blackwell Publishing, Oxford.

Maughan RJ (2002) Food and fluid intake during exercise. *Canadian Journal of Applied Physiology* **26**: S71–S78.

Proulx CI, Ducharme MB & Kenny GP (2003) Effect of water temperature on cooling efficiency during hyperthermia in humans. *Journal of Applied Physiology* **94**: 1317–23.

Wasserman K, Hansen JE, Sue DY, Casaburi R & Whipp BJ (1999) *Principles of Exercise Testing and Interpretation*, 3rd edition. Lippincott Williams & Wilkins, Philadelphia.

Crash trauma and blood loss

CASE AND MCQS

Case introduction

It is the middle of summer in Australia and the temperature is about 30°C.

A man (P.T.), age 53, is brought to the hospital by ambulance at 10.00 hours. He was found at 09.00 hours in his car which had crashed into a tree at the side of the road. He had lost blood from lesions to his legs and his legs had been trapped in the car.

The time of the accident was not clear but was probably between 6 and 12 hours previously. The patient is semi-comatose and confused and it was difficult to obtain a history at the crash site. The ambulance officers report that there appeared to have been about a litre of blood lost.
On examination, there are abrasions to the forehead that have stopped bleeding. There is a laceration on the left thigh caused by broken glass and contusion and bruising of both thighs. The patient is tender over the abdomen, particularly in the left upper quadrant. He is confused and smells of alcohol (information is obtained later that he had been drinking at the local country hotel and had left there about 22.00 hours). His extremities are cold and sweaty. No other localizing signs are found.

Blood pressure is 90/60 mmHg; pulse rate 130 beats/min; respiratory rate 14/min.

An electrocardiogram is taken which, apart from the tachycardia, appears normal. Blood is taken for haematology and biochemistry and a drip is inserted into a forearm vein.

Q1 Assume that prior to the accident Mr T.'s haematology was normal, with haemoglobin (Hb) 15.5 g/dl, haematocrit (Hct) 43% and plasma albumin of 36 g/litre. Which of the following is most likely to be the result of his haematological examination on admission?

A. Hb 15, Hct 45, albumin 36
B. Hb 10, Hct 30, albumin 32
C. Hb 12, Hct 35, albumin 28
D. Hb 15, Hct 35, albumin 36
E. Hb 10, Hct 35, albumin 32

Q2 Mr T. has apparently lost only around 1 litre of blood. This would not be sufficient to cause the degree of hypotension and tachycardia that exists. What other avenues of blood loss may be involved?

A. loss of blood into the thigh muscles
B. extravasation of plasma into the damaged muscle
C. loss of blood into the abdomen
D. either A and C
E. any of A, B and C

Q3 If there is loss of blood into the peritoneal cavity, from which of the following structures is the bleeding most likely to originate?

A. liver
B. spleen
C. kidneys
D. liver and kidneys
E. spleen and kidneys

Q4 Typical normal values (mmol/l) for plasma biochemistry are sodium 140, potassium 4.0, creatinine 0.08, urea 6.0. Which of the following combinations of values is most likely to represent Mr T.'s situation at present?

A. sodium 140, potassium 4.0, creatinine 0.08, urea 6.0
B. sodium 150, potassium 5.0, creatinine 0.12, urea 5.0
C. sodium 130, potassium 3.5, creatinine 0.15, urea 8.0
D. sodium 145, potassium 4.5, creatinine 0.10, urea 8.0
E. sodium 150, potassium 5.5, creatinine 0.15, urea 8.0

Q5 Which of the following fluids and volume would be most appropriate to give Mr T. intravenously as a matter of urgency?

A. whole blood – 1 litre over 4 hours
B. normal saline – 1 litre over 4 hours
C. fresh frozen plasma – 1 litre over 4 hours
D. 5% glucose in distilled water – 1 litre over 4 hours
E. normal saline – 1 litre immediately, then 1 litre/hour

A drip is set up and an infusion started. Blood is taken for cross-matching to obtain appropriate blood for transfusion. The results of the biochemistry come back and reveal the following:

Haemoglobin	12.1 g/dl
Haematocrit	35%
Albumin	28 g/l
Sodium	145 mmol/l
Potassium	4.5 mmol/l
Creatinine	0.10 mmol/l
Urea	8.0 mmol/l

Ultrasound shows a haematoma on the spleen, with no obvious tear.

At the time of initial examination it was noted that Mr T. had not passed urine since removal from the crash site. His bladder is catheterized and is found to contain 400 ml of urine that is discoloured and on testing is found to contain some myoglobin, probably due to the damage to his thigh muscles. The catheter is left indwelling and an hour later he has passed 25 ml of urine. This is a very low rate of urine formation (*oliguria*) by comparison with the value of 70–100 ml/h expected in a normal, hydrated individual.

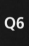 **Q6** Which one of the following compositions of urine passed in this hour would suggest that the oliguria is reversible? (solute values in mmol/l, osmolality in mosmol/l)

A. sodium 25, osmol 500, creatinine 6, urea 300
B. sodium 85, osmol 310, creatinine 0.6, urea 30
C. sodium 25, osmol 200, creatinine 6, urea 30
D. sodium 55, osmol 400, creatinine 2, urea 100
E. sodium 55, osmol 200, creatinine 0.6, urea 30

 Q7 Which of the above urine compositions would suggest that this person has developed acute tubular necrosis?

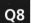 **Q8** In acute tubular necrosis, which segment of the nephron is the most susceptible to damage?

A. proximal tubule 1st part
B. proximal tubule 2nd part
C. thick ascending limb of loop of Henle
D. cortical collecting system
E. medullary collecting system

 Q9 Acute tubular necrosis results from an extension of the normal physiological responses to a low plasma volume and pressure. Which one of the following statements related to these mechanisms is *incorrect*?

A. a low sodium chloride concentration at the macula densa increases renin secretion
B. the efferent arteriole is more sensitive than the afferent arteriole to angiotensin II
C. tubulo-glomerular feedback is mediated by dilatation of the afferent arteriole
D. a low sodium chloride concentration at the macula densa causes dilatation of the afferent arteriole
E. renin and angiotensin II are important mediators of tubulo-glomerular feedback

Mr T. is given 3 litres of saline intravenously over 2 hours and his blood pressure rises. He is then given 1 litre of blood: his blood pressure increases to 120/80 mmHg and his pulse rate falls to 80 beats/min. He becomes less confused and confirms that he had been drinking the previous night and that he had probably crashed at about 23.00 hours – that is, 10 hours before he was found. However, despite the rise in blood pressure and better tissue perfusion, his urine output is still low.

Q10 Assuming he receives *no further fluid supplements*, which of the following changes in plasma composition is *least* likely to occur over the next 4 hours?

A. creatinine will rise
B. potassium will rise
C. sodium will rise
D. urea will rise.
E. pH will fall

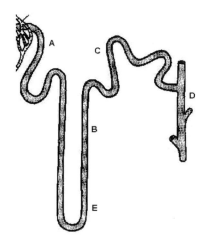

Fig. 18.1 A nephron.

Figure 18.1 shows a nephron, with five segments labelled as follows:
A. proximal tubule
B. thick ascending limb of loop of Henle
C. distal tubule
D. collecting system
E. thin ascending limb of loop of Henle

Q11 In which segment is there the greatest secretion of H⁺?

Q12 In which segment is most potassium absorbed?

Q13 In which segment is the concentration of potassium lowest?

Q14 In which segment is most potassium secreted?

Q15 In which segment do thiazide diuretics act?

Q16 In which segment is permeability to water increased in the presence of antidiuretic hormone (ADH)?

Q17 In which segment is sodium transport increased in the presence of ADH?

Over the next 4 hours Mr T.'s urine output stays low and has the following composition:

Sodium	85 mmol/l
Osmolality	300 mosmol/l
Creatinine	0.4 mmol/l
Urea	25 mmol/l

The urine is dark and contains myoglobin. Plasma electrolytes at 16.00 hours (about 18 hours after the accident) are:

Sodium	140 mmol/l
Potassium	5.7 mmol/l
Creatinine	0.15 mmol/l
Urea	16 mmol/l

His arterial acid-base status is assessed. Normal values are:

Bicarbonate (HCO_3^-)	22–28 mmol/l
$P\text{CO}_2$	35–45 mmHg
pH	7.35–7.45

Q18 Which of the following is most likely to be found in this man?

A. HCO_3^- 30, $P\text{CO}_2$ 48.0, pH 7.5
B. HCO_3^- 25, $P\text{CO}_2$ 41.7, pH 7.4
C. HCO_3^- 25, $P\text{CO}_2$ 43.0, pH 7.3
D. HCO_3^- 18, $P\text{CO}_2$ 30.0, pH 7.3
E. HCO_3^- 18, $P\text{CO}_2$ 36.0, pH 7.2

In view of these values and the rise in potassium, it is decided to add sodium bicarbonate to the intravenous fluid. Blood pressure has stabilized and tissue perfusion is good, so the rapid infusion of fluids is stopped and a diagnosis is made at this time of acute tubular necrosis due to hypotension and myoglobinuria.

Q19 All of the following can kill a person with acute tubular necrosis. Which one of the following is most likely to kill this patient if not treated?

A. sodium retention and high blood pressure
B. high plasma potassium
C. low plasma pH
D. retention of nitrogenous products
E. water overload

Q20 What has contributed to the rapid rise in potassium in this patient?

A. breakdown of muscle cells
B. haemolysis of blood
C. acidosis
D. both A and B
E. all of A, B and C

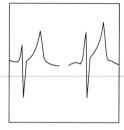

 Q21 In a person with acute tubular necrosis, which of the following is the usual outcome?

A. chronic renal failure always results
B. there is always recovery
C. patients usually require dialysis before recovery occurs
D. patients usually require permanent dialysis
E. severe dietary restriction is essential

Mr T. remains oliguric, passing about 25 ml/h urine with a similar composition to that recorded previously.

 Q22 Assuming no fluid intake by mouth, which one of the following orders for intravenous fluid over the next 24 hours do you consider most appropriate?

A. 500 ml of normal saline
B. 500 ml of 5% glucose in distilled water
C. 1000 ml of normal saline
D. 1000 ml of 5% glucose in distilled water
E. 2000 ml of 5% glucose in distilled water

As well as this intravenous fluid, 200 mg of the diuretic furosemide is given intravenously. Urine output increases over the next 3 hours to 45 ml/h but then returns to its previous level.

Plasma biochemistry the next day, approximately 36 hours after the accident, is:

Sodium	135 mmol/l
Potassium	6.6 mmol/l
Bicarbonate	15 mmol/l
Creatinine	0.24 mmol/l
Urea	26 mmol/l

Blood pressure is 130/85 mmHg; pulse rate is 70 beats/min.

An ECG shows tall peaked T waves particularly in the precordial leads (Fig. 18.2). These peaked T waves could occur in a normal individual but, since they were not present at admission, they suggest an effect of the high plasma potassium on the heart. If not treated, these changes would progress to cardiac arrhythmia.

Fig. 18.2 ECG recording (thoracic leads V$_3$ and V$_4$) taken from Mr T. 36 hours after his accident.

Q23 Which one of the following would be *least* useful for reducing the likelihood of hyperkalaemic cardiac arrhythmia?

A. intravenous glucose and insulin
B. intravenous sodium bicarbonate
C. oral cation-exchange resin
D. peritoneal dialysis
E. intravenous furosemide

Mr T. is treated as discussed in the answer to Question 23 and his plasma potassium falls to 5.9 mmol/l.

Daily peritoneal dialysis is continued over the next 8 days with appropriate adjustments to his electrolyte balance. On the 11th day post accident he starts to pass a large amount of urine (polyuria) and dialysis is stopped. The polyuria continues for the next 3 days then returns to a more normal urine output.

At discharge from hospital, 14 days after the accident, plasma biochemistry shows:

Sodium	140 mmol/l
Potassium	3.6 mmol/l
Bicarbonate	24 mmol/l
Creatinine	0.11 mmol/l
Urea	7.5 mmol/l

MCQ ANSWERS AND FEEDBACK

1.C. Blood loss causes precapillary vasoconstriction; this reduces intracapillary hydrostatic pressure and so interstitial water enters the bloodstream. Thus, Hct and HB fall in proportion. Albumin must also fall to the same extent, at least, but may fall even more if there is extravasation of plasma into damaged tissue. Answer C is the only one to show this combination.

2.E. From the history, external loss of blood, bleeding into thigh muscle, bleeding into abdomen and extravasation of plasma into damaged muscles may all have taken place.

3.B. The kidneys are retroperitoneal and so renal bleeding is usually retroperitoneal. The spleen is more susceptible to damage and bleeding than the liver and so splenic bleeding is the most likely cause of bleeding into the peritoneal cavity after trauma.

4.D. The sodium should be in the normal range, that is, A or D. Potassium would be normal or slightly elevated, as in A, B, D or E. Creatinine and urea would both rise as the excretion of both depends on glomerular filtration.

5.E. The important thing is immediately to replace fluid and electrolytes. One litre of saline should be given rapidly, followed by a continuing infusion. Blood will probably also be needed as the falls in Hb and Hct may have underestimated total loss, but that requires cross-matching and some time. It would be wrong to wait until this information is available. Even if blood were available immediately, it is important to correct the situation rapidly, not over 4 hours.

6.A. The renal damage is potentially reversible if filtration is continuing and the reabsorptive processes for sodium and water are intact. Remember that, normally, about 99% of water is reabsorbed (so urinary creatinine is about 100 times that of plasma) and 99.9% of sodium is reabsorbed. Thus the criteria for reversible oliguria are low urine sodium, urine osmolality higher than plasma and both urea and creatinine many times the plasma values, indicating that intense water reabsorption is taking place.

7.B. Creatinine and urea are less than 10 times plasma concentration. Sodium is 85 mmol and the osmolarity is close to that of plasma. This indicates impairment of selective tubular reabsorption. Results C and E are very unlikely ever to occur. Result D is indeterminate; a patient with these values could either go on to acute tubular necrosis or have reversible oliguria.

8.C. The thick ascending limb of Henle's loop is most susceptible to damage as it is in a region of relatively poor blood supply and has a very high turnover of ATP. Damage to the proximal tubule follows soon after.

9.E. The first four statements are all correct. However, the renin–angiotensin system does not mediate tubulo-glomerular feedback. The afferent arteriole tone alterations that constitute this are controlled by nitric oxide, adenosine and prostaglandins.

10.C. Sodium concentration is unlikely to rise as sodium and water are reabsorbed together. However, impaired renal function will lead to a rise in creatinine, urea, H^+ (that is, pH will fall) and potassium. The rises in H^+ and potassium are due to continuing production of acidic metabolites and to release of intracellular potassium under acid conditions.

11.A. H^+ is secreted in large amounts in the proximal tubules to absorb sodium and bicarbonate. None of this H^+ is lost in the urine. A smaller amount of H^+ is secreted in the distal nephrons but, after bicarbonate has been absorbed, this H^+ is excreted in the urine as titratable acidity, NH_4^+ and a little free H^+.

12.A. The greatest amount of potassium is absorbed in the proximal tubule.

13.B. A large amount of the filtered potassium has already been reabsorbed in the proximal tubule and most of that remaining is reabsorbed during its passage through the loop.

14.D. Potassium is secreted mostly in the collecting system down an electrochemical gradient produced by sodium reabsorption.

15.C. Thiazide diuretics bind to the sodium/chloride cotransporter in the cortical diluting segment of the early distal nephron.

16.D. ADH increases the water permeability of the collecting system in both the cortex and the medulla. This effect is mediated by increasing cyclic AMP production inside the cells, causing aquaporins to be inserted into the luminal membrane.

17.B. ADH increases sodium transport in the thick ascending limb of the loop of Henle. It also affects potassium permeability in the collecting system. In the absence of ADH, the collecting system is relatively impermeable to potassium.

18.D. Renal failure has started, as indicted by the rise of creatinine to 0.15 mmol/l. Under these circumstances H^+ will have been retained, stimulating the reaction $H^+ + HCO_3^- \rightarrow H_2O + CO_2$, so plasma bicarbonate will fall (answers D or E). Respiratory compensation will take place, causing P_{CO_2} to fall in approximately the same proportion and thus minimizing the fall in pH, so the answer must be D. Remember also that the conditions of the Henderson–Hasselbalch equation must be maintained:

$$pH = 6.1 + \log HCO_3^-/(0.03 \times P_{CO_2})$$

This is fulfilled by A, B and D but not by C or E. However, in A and B there is no retention of H^+.

19.B. A rapid rise in plasma potassium is likely to cause alterations in cardiac conduction, arrhythmias and death.

20.E. Breakdown of damaged muscle cells, haemolysis of red blood cells in the damaged tissues and the outward shift of intracellular potassium associated with acidosis will all elevate plasma potassium.

21.C. Most people with acute tubular necrosis from this cause will recover. Historically, severe dietary restriction of protein and sodium intake was used, but it is usual now to have moderate dietary restrictions and to initiate dialysis early.

22.D. Mr T. is not excreting a significant amount of sodium but you need to replace the fluid losses. These consist of urine, about 500 ml or less (but measure it) and losses due to respiration and insensible perspiration, minus the water of metabolism. The total loss would usually be about 1000 ml, which should be given as 5% glucose in distilled water.

23.E. Correction of acidosis with sodium bicarbonate will move potassium back into the cells. This would be aided by glucose and insulin, which causes glucose uptake into the liver and concomitant movement of potassium into the cells. A cation exchange resin such as resonium A would prevent potassium absorption from the gut, but is slow to act. Peritoneal dialysis will remove potassium from the body. Thus these four approaches are all useful. Intravenous furosemide may increase urine output but would not be a reliable way to reduce potassium levels.

CASE REVIEW

This man has been involved in an accident and has had some blood loss and trauma to his legs. His clinical condition is worse than would occur with the loss of 1 litre of blood and there is almost certainly internal bleeding and extravasation of blood into his thighs and possibly into his peritoneal cavity. The haematocrit, haemoglobin and albumen would fall by a similar percentage as whole blood is lost. If he has blood loss into the peritoneal cavity, it is most likely to be from the spleen, since bleeding from the kidneys is usually retroperitoneal.

Over a 12-hour period, there would be little alteration in plasma biochemistry and most values would be close to the normal range. This person should have a drip set up and be given saline rapidly while cross-matching blood, which he will also require.

The problem in such a case is that the patient may develop acute renal tubular necrosis. There are two major contributing factors. The first is severe hypotension and shock. The second is a possible crush injury to the legs that will cause release of myoglobin into the blood. Myoglobin is toxic to the kidneys.

If a person has severe hypotension, the composition of the urine can enable us to determine whether the low urine output is a physiological response to hypotension or whether acute tubular necrosis has occurred. Reversible oliguria and acute tubular necrosis can be differentiated as follows:
- Oliguria – less than 30 ml/h
- Acute tubular necrosis – damage to tubules leading to un-selective reabsorption
- Pre-renal failure – low blood pressure and volume deple-tion lead to intense salt and water reabsorption.

Electrolyte problems associated with acute renal failure are:
- Na^+ retention $\rightarrow$ high BP $\rightarrow$ pulmonary oedema $\rightarrow$ death
- K^+ retention $\rightarrow$ high plasma K^+ $\rightarrow$ cardiac arrhythmia $\rightarrow$ death
- H^+ retention $\rightarrow$ acidosis $\rightarrow$ K^+ out of cells.

When the response is physiological and the kidney has not developed acute tubular necrosis, there will be intense sodium and water reabsorption stimulated by the low blood pressure, with increased vasopressin (ADH), angiotensin II and aldosterone release. Thus urine volume is low (due to ADH), the urine sodium concentration is low (due to angiotensin II and aldosterone), osmolality will be greater than that of plasma, and creatinine and urea concentrations will be much higher than in plasma.

By contrast, if acute tubular necrosis has developed, then the composition of the urine will approach that of plasma as sodium and water can no longer be selectively absorbed. There is clearly some overlap as there is a transition between the two states.

When blood pressure falls, this activates tubulo-glomerular feedback, causing dilatation of the afferent arteriole (proba-bly due to release of NO, adenosine and prostaglandins) in an attempt to maintain glomerular filtration rate (GFR) despite a low perfusion pressure. The low blood pressure will also cause renin release, which increases circulating angiotensin II. The efferent arteriole is more sensitive than the afferent arteriole to angiotension and thus there is efferent arteriole vasoconstriction, which will also maintain GFR by increasing the filtration fraction (Fig. 18.3). The sequence of events in tubulo-glomerular feedback is as follows:
- Individual GFR tends to stay constant
- Macula densa senses Na^+Cl^-
- Low Na^+ causes local vasodilators release
- Local vasodilators: adenosine, NO, prostaglandins
- Vasodilate afferent arteriole
- Increases GFR
- Corrects low Na^+ at macula densa.

If, however, the low pressure persists, the circulating angi-otensin II level becomes so high that, together with activation of the sympathetic nerves, it causes afferent arteriolar vaso-

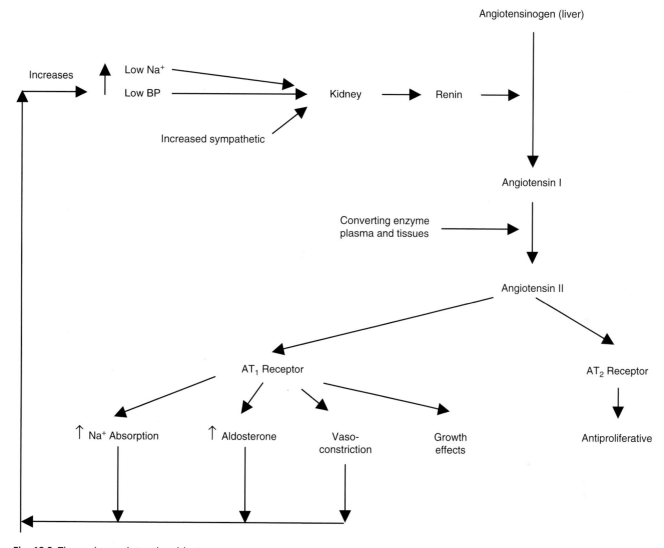

Fig. 18.3 The renin–angiotensin–aldosterone system.

constriction and leads to a reduction in GFR. The tubular structures with the greatest oxygen demand (thick ascending limb of the loop of Henle) are damaged first, followed by the proximal tubular cells. Theoretically (and occasionally in practice), impairment of tubular function should cause polyuria, but usually there is unselective reabsorption of filtrate, just as in a capillary.

Patients who progress to acute tubular necrosis will start to accumulate substances that are normally excreted from their plasma. As water and sodium are both retained, the plasma sodium concentration usually stays the same. However, the retention of sodium and water will lead to blood pressure elevation. Protons are produced by metabolism of both dietary and body protein, and in a person on an omnivore diet there is about 50 mmol/day of H^+ to be excreted. Thus with renal functional impairment, H^+ will accumulate in plasma

and acidosis will develop, although it will be compensated by respiratory adjustments. The present patient's blood showed a pH that was low but not excessively so. The main finding was a low plasma bicarbonate and a low $Paco_2$ due to respiratory compensation which blows off CO_2, thus reducing the variation in pH.

Even though no potassium may be taken in by mouth, normal cell metabolism will cause potassium to increase. In addition, breakdown of damaged muscle cells will lead to a rise in potassium and acidosis will also cause potassium to move out of cells into plasma. The potassium in urine comes from secretion in the collecting system and, if this transport is impaired, urinary potassium will be low. It is the rise in plasma potassium that is most likely to rapidly kill a patient with impaired tubular function and needs to be prevented (Table 18.1).

Table 18.1 Effects of disturbed plasma potassium and calcium on the ECG

Hyperkalaemia – progressively as plasma K+ rises	Tall peaked T waves
	Flattening of P waves
	Prolongation of PR interval
	Atrial standstill
	Widening of QRS complex
	Sine wave of QRS and T waves
	Death
Hypokalaemia	Flat T waves
	Prominent U waves
	Ventricular arrhythmias
Hypercalcaemia	Prolongation of ST segment
	May be confused with hypokalaemia

The most useful method for acutely reducing plasma potassium is to correct the acidosis with sodium bicarbonate, but this may increase the sodium load. Glucose and insulin administered together will cause the liver to take up glucose and potassium enters the liver cells in parallel. Potassium absorption from the gut can also be prevented by cation exchange resins such as resonium A and plasma potassium can be lowered by dialysis.

Most patients with this type of presentation will require dialysis, although some will recover without it. The principles of management are to prevent death from high potassium and acidosis by the actions mentioned above, and to prevent hypertension and pulmonary oedema by restriction of sodium and water intake.

KEY POINTS

- The amount of blood loss is frequently much greater than the external appearance due to internal bleeding.
- Following blood loss the kidney avidly reabsorbs sodium and water.
- After severe hypotension and crush damage to muscles, acute tubular necrosis may result.
- In acute renal failure, retention of potassium, sodium, water and protons causes acute problems.
- Potassium retention with hyperkalaemia causes disturbance in cardiac conduction leading to death.

ADDITIONAL READING

Seldin DW & Giebisch G (2000) *The Kidney: Physiology and Pathophysiology*, 3rd edition. Lippincott Williams & Wilkins, Philadelphia.

Rose BD & Post TW (2001) *Clinical Physiology of Acid Base and Electrolyte Disorders*, 5th edition. McGraw-Hill, New York.

Souhami RL & Moxham T (2002) *Textbook of Medicine*, 4th edition. Churchill Livingstone, London.

Whitworth JA & Lawrence JR (1994) *Textbook of Renal Disease*, 2nd edition. Churchill Livingstone, London.

Braunwald E *et al.* (2001) *Harrison's Principles of Internal Medicine*, 15th edition. McGraw-Hill, New York.

Weakness, weight gain and bruising

CASE AND MCQS

Case introduction

Ms J.H., a 33-year-old woman who has had two children, now aged 9 and 7, presents with a history of fatigue and muscle weakness. These symptoms have been present for the last 3 years but have recently been getting worse. She also states that she has gained weight and has started to bruise easily.

She has no history of past illnesses and her pregnancies had caused no problems.

On examination, the patient is obese, particularly on the trunk, and has a hump-like swelling on her back. Her limbs are relatively slender except for some slight ankle oedema. There are some purple streaks (striae) across her abdomen and buttocks. Her blood pressure is 175/105 mmHg.

A clinical diagnosis is made that Ms H. has Cushing's disease or Cushing's syndrome, most likely due to excessive levels of cortisol in her blood. You schedule a variety of biochemical and radiological tests to confirm this diagnosis.

Q1 Cushing's syndrome could be caused by:

A. excessive secretion of adrenocorticotrophic hormone (ACTH)
B. excessive secretion of cortisol
C. failure to break down cortisol
D. either A or B
E. any of A, B or C

Q2 Assuming normal plasma values (sodium 139 mmol/l, potassium 4.2 mmol/l, chloride 101 mmol/l, bicarbonate 27 mmol/l), which of the biochemical results listed in Table 19.1 would be most likely to be associated with Cushing's syndrome?

Q3 Which of the following can cause cortisol hypersecretion?

A. tumour of the adrenal medulla
B. tumour of the adrenal cortex
C. tumour of the pituitary gland
D. carcinoid tumour
E. either B, C or D

Table 19.1 Options for Question 2

	Sodium (mmol/l)	Potassium (mmol/l)	Chloride (mmol/l)	Bicarbonate (mmol/l)
A	145	4.2	106	25
B	145	3.2	95	37
C	139	4.2	101	27
D	135	3.2	95	34
E	135	4.5	101	25

Q4 A CAT scan of the abdomen reveals that both Ms H.'s adrenal glands are enlarged. Which one of the alternatives in Question 3 is most likely to be associated with bilateral adrenal gland enlargement?

Q5 The anterior pituitary is the source of several hormones in addition to ACTH. Which one of the following hormones is *not* secreted by the anterior pituitary?

A. follicle-stimulating hormone
B. thyroid-stimulating hormone
C. parathyroid-stimulating hormone
D. growth hormone
E. prolactin

Q6 Draw a diagram indicating the relationship between the hypothalamus, the anterior pituitary and the posterior pituitary.

Q7 What cell types exist in the anterior pituitary and what does each secrete?

Q8 The secretion of ACTH is influenced by:

A. circulating cortisol levels
B. corticotrophin-releasing factor secreted by the hypothalamus
C. neuroendocrine reflexes
D. both A and B
E. all of A, B and C

Q9 Which of the following is *not* an effect of cortisol?

A. increased gluconeogenesis by the liver
B. increased glycogen synthesis by the liver
C. increased protein synthesis by striated muscle
D. decreased glucose uptake by adipose tissue
E. increased lipid mobilization from adipose tissue

Q10 Which of the following statements is *not* correct in relation to control of growth hormone secretion?

A. its release is inhibited by somatostatin
B. its release is stimulated by deep sleep
C. its release is stimulated by stress
D. its release is stimulated by a low blood glucose
E. its release is stimulated by REM sleep

Q11 Release of growth hormone produces all of the following effects *except*:

A. increased protein formation by muscle
B. increased glucose uptake by muscle
C. increased glucose formation by the liver
D. increased somatomedin production by the liver
E. increased lipolysis by adipose tissue

Q12  Which of the following hormones act directly on tissues without the need to stimulate secretion of a second hormone from an endocrine gland?

A. ACTH
B. prolactin
C. thyroid-stimulating hormone
D. luteinizing hormone
E. both B and D

Q13 Which of the following pituitary hormones are important to the mother around the time of birth?

A. luteinizing hormone
B. oxytocin
C. prolactin
D. both A and B
E. both B and C

The results of Ms H.'s tests are returned.
- CT scanning shows bilateral adrenal hypertrophy.
- X-ray of the pituitary fossa shows no enlargement.
- Cortisol levels in the plasma and the urine are elevated.
- There is no diurnal variation of cortisol levels.
- Plasma cortisol is not suppressed by a standard dose of the synthetic glucocorticoid dexamethasone but is suppressed by a high dose.

A diagnosis is made that Ms H. has Cushing's disease due to hypersecretion of ACTH by the corticotropes of the anterior pituitary.

Q14 How would you further confirm that the problem is a primary dysfunction of the pituitary gland?

Q15 What is the most common cause of Cushing's syndrome in our community?

A. adrenal tumours
B. pituitary hypersecretion
C. liver disease
D. bilateral adrenal hypertrophy
E. administration of steroid therapy

Investigations are performed which imply that Ms H. has microadenomata of the anterior pituitary. These are removed by transphenoidal surgery.

She makes a good recovery. Twelve months later, she is normotensive and has lost the physical features of Cushing's syndrome.

MCQ ANSWERS AND FEEDBACK

1.E. Cushing's syndrome reflects an excessive plasma level of cortisol. This can result from excessive secretion of ACTH by the anterior pituitary stimulating excessive synthesis and secretion of cortisol from the adrenal gland. It can also occur if there is a failure to break down cortisol, for instance because of liver disease.

2.D. Excess plasma levels of cortisol have many effects on the body that lead to elevated blood pressure. The high level of cortisol means that the mineralocorticoid receptors (normally activated by aldosterone) are stimulated leading to sodium and water retention. This also causes potassium loss by the kidney, as well as causing H^+ excretion, with consequent elevation of bicarbonate. Cortisol also has an effect on water metabolism and when it is in high amounts free water clearance is impaired, either by an effect on responsiveness of the collecting system to ADH or a central effect on ADH release. Thus in a patient with high plasma cortisol, plasma potassium would be low, bicarbonate would be high (answers B or D) and sodium would be low (answer D).

3.E. Cortisol is not secreted by the adrenal medulla. Tumours of the adrenal medulla secrete catecholamines, which may cause severe episodic hypertension (*phaeochromocytoma*). Cortisol can be secreted by tumours of the adrenal cortex. In addition, carcinoid tumours and tumours of the anterior pituitary (which may be very small) secrete ACTH that stimulates the adrenals to hypersecrete cortisol.

4.C. Since ACTH acts systemically, excessive secretion of ACTH will result in both adrenals being enlarged. Both adrenals would also be enlarged with carcinoid tumours but anterior pituitary overactivity is more common.

5.C. The anterior pituitary controls the function of a number of endocrine glands in the gonads, the adrenal cortex and the thyroid. However, the parathyroid gland has no regulatory hormone released by the anterior pituitary.

6. The anterior pituitary is connected to the hypothalamus by a venous portal system (see Fig. 19.1). The posterior pituitary is part of the brain and contains axons that have their cell bodies in the supraoptic and paraventricular nuclei of the hypothalamus.

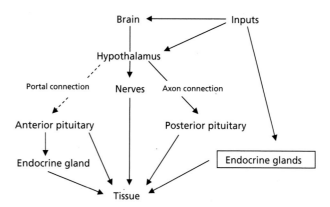

**INTEGRATION OF RESPONSES
NEURAL AND HORMONAL**

Fig. 19.1 A schematic diagram indicating the interaction between the nervous and endocrine systems.

A key role is played by the hypothalamus, which contains receptors monitoring a number of plasma parameters, e.g. osmolality and temperature. In addition, both peripheral and central nervous systems impact on this structure. The hypothalamus releases factors into the portal blood, which travel directly to the anterior pituitary and control the release of various anterior pituitary hormones. There are both stimulatory and inhibitory hypothalamic factors. Most of the anterior pituitary hormones act by stimulating secretion of other hormones from peripheral endocrine glands. By contrast, growth hormones and prolactin have direct effects on their target tissues, as is also the case for the hormones released from the posterior pituitary – oxytocin and vasopressin (ADH).

7. The cell types used to be classified as basophilic and acidophilic. They are now classified according to their hormone secretion. The types, their frequency and their secretions are:
- Somatotropes – 50% total, secrete growth hormone
- Corticotropes – 20% total, secrete ACTH
- Thyrotropes – 5% total, secrete thyroid-stimulating hormone (TSH)
- Lactotropes – 20% total, secrete prolactin
- Gonadotropes – 5% total, secrete luteinizing hormone (LH) and follicle-stimulating hormone (FSH).

8.E. The secretion of ACTH by the anterior pituitary is stimulated by corticotrophin-releasing factor (CRF) secreted by the hypothalamus. Neural inputs to the central nervous system associated with stress stimulate CRF release. Circulating cortisol both reduces the sensitivity of the corticotropes to CRF and inhibits secretion of CRF from the hypothalamus.

9.C. Cortisol has a large number of metabolic effects. It increases formation of glucose in the liver by stimulating protein gluconeogenesis and increases glycogen synthesis. Glucose uptake by adipose tissue is decreased and lipids are mobilized from adipose tissue. In the plasma, the glucose level is frequently elevated. Cortisol increases production of a large number of proteins that are involved in cellular regulatory pathways. In muscle cells, however, the effect is an increased breakdown and decreased synthesis of muscle proteins, leading to wasting of skeletal muscles.

10.E. The secretion of growth hormone exhibits a circadian rhythm with the greatest secretion during deep sleep. REM (rapid eye movement) sleep reduces its secretion. A similar response is seen with secretion of renin by the kidney. Growth hormone secretion is stimulated by growth hormone-releasing factor and is inhibited by somatostatin released from different hypothalamic nuclei. Stress and low blood glucose stimulate growth hormone secretion by effects exerted through the hypothalamus.

11.B. Growth hormone has direct effects on most tissues of the body but these are complemented by an increased formation of somatomedin by the liver, which stimulates cell proliferation and growth in bone (leading to increased linear growth in the young) and to increased protein synthesis in many organs. Growth hormone directly stimulates gluconeogenesis by the liver and increases protein formation by muscles (anabolism).

It increases lipolysis and thus reduces adipose tissue. It also decreases glucose uptake into both adipose and muscle tissue.

12.B. Prolactin secreted by the lactotropes of the anterior pituitary has a direct effect on mammary tissue. ACTH and TSH both act on their target glands to increase synthesis and secretion of cortisol and thyroxine respectively. Luteinizing hormone acts on the ovary to stimulate the secretion of progesterone (predominantly) and also some oestrogens.

13.E. Oxytocin is formed in the hypothalamus but stored and secreted from the posterior pituitary. It causes contraction of many smooth muscle cells around the body. By causing contraction of the bladder it may stimulate micturition. At the time of birth, it causes uterine contraction. Oxytocin is, however, of particular importance in lactation, aiding the transfer of milk from the alveoli to the larger milk ducts.

Prolactin stimulates milk synthesis by the breast tissue. Its release is stimulated by suckling, thus providing a stimulus for milk synthesis prior to the next feed. Prolactin inhibits the secretion of gonadotrope-releasing factor from the hypothalamus and thus people are less likely to become pregnant (but still can) while an infant is breastfeeding.

14. It is possible to collect blood from the inferior petrosal sinus on both sides and measure ACTH levels, thus verifying that there is hypersecretion from the pituitary and also identifying the side from which it is secreted.

15.E. The most common cause of Cushing's syndrome in Western communities is the administration of glucocorticoids as anti-inflammatory and immunosuppressant drugs in a wide range of clinical situations. These include asthma, rheumatoid arthritis, nephrotic syndrome, post-organ transplant and many others.

CASE REVIEW

Cushing's syndrome is due to excessive amounts of glucocorticoids, principally cortisol, in the body. Cortisol is secreted from the zona fasciculata of the adrenal gland and its synthesis and secretion are stimulated by anterior pituitary release of ACTH. Secretion of ACTH from the corticotrope cells is stimulated by the release of corticotrophin-releasing factor from the hypothalamus. This travels to the anterior pituitary gland by a portal system (Fig. 19.1). The release of corticotrophin-releasing factor is in turn controlled by negative feedback of cortisol on its secretion and by input from the central nervous system. In addition, cortisol has a direct action on the corticotrope cells of the anterior pituitary, reducing their sensitivity to corticotrophin-releasing factor.

Cortisol is an exceedingly important hormone in maintaining normal body function and has actions on most cells of the body. Cortisol crosses the cell membrane and binds to cytoplasmic receptors. These are then internalized into the nucleus, with stimulation of synthesis of a large number of proteins. The main features of cortisol under physiological conditions are:
- Released in response to many types of stress including trauma, infection, extreme temperatures, cerebral arousal

- Has a 'permissive' action for mineralocorticoid hormones
- Promotes muscle protein breakdown (*catabolism*)
- Increases gluconeogenesis
- Increases lipid mobilization
- Has anti-inflammatory effects
- Has immunosuppressive effects.

In adipose tissue, cortisol increases lipid mobilization. It also increases hepatic gluconeogenesis, increases glycogen synthesis and reduces cellular uptake of glucose. As a result, plasma glucose rises. In muscle tissue there is decreased protein synthesis and increased protein degradation. In the kidneys, by acting on mineralocorticoid receptors, cortisol increases sodium retention and causes potassium and H^+ loss. It also reduces free water secretion and thus plasma sodium and potassium are both decreased while pH and bicarbonate are increased.

Cortisol and related synthetic glucocorticoids (for instance cortisone, prednisolone, dexamethasone) also have important anti-inflammatory effects and this is of critical importance in the treatment of many diseases. The prevention and reversal of inflammation is mediated by stabilization of cell membranes, so limiting release of proinflammatory mediators, and by suppression of T cell production. These actions of glucocorticoids make them life-saving medicines in conditions such as allergic shock and when immune suppression is necessary for survival of organ transplants, and valuable for treatment of inflammatory rheumatic conditions.

Under circumstances of abnormally high circulating levels of cortisol or other glucocorticoids, the multiple actions that they have on body cells are reflected in the wide range of clinical consequences. These include hypertension, muscle weakness, fatigue, central adiposity, purple striae on the skin, osteoporosis, diabetes, psychiatric disorders, susceptibility to infection and many others.

Plasma glucocorticoid levels may be high due to therapeutic administration of a synthetic cortisol analogue or because of hypersecretion from an adrenal cortical tumour (relatively uncommon). In these situations, plasma ACTH will be low due to negative feedback on ACTH production. Alternatively, there may be cortisol hypersecretion due to hypersecretion of ACTH from carcinoid tumours or from small adenomata in the anterior pituitary gland. When there is hypersecretion from the anterior pituitary, this is known as *Cushing's disease*.

Blood can be collected from the inferior petrosal sinus on both sides and ACTH levels measured. This will confirm that there is hypersecretion from the pituitary and not from a carcinoid and it will also localize the side, which will aid in the surgical therapy. Various suppression tests can be done with dexamethasone to try to distinguish between carcinoid tumour secretion and anterior pituitary secretion but these are not as definitive.

As might be predicted from its multiple cellular effects, lack of cortisol also results in dysfunction of multiple body systems. This syndrome is termed Addison's disease (*chronic adrenocortical insufficiency*). Some of its features are:
- Low plasma sodium
- High plasma potassium
- Acidosis
- Low blood pressure
- Low blood glucose
- Muscle weakness
- Skin pigmentation.

KEY POINTS

- The release of ACTH and other hormones by the anterior pituitary is controlled by factors secreted by the hypothalamus.
- The hypothalamus and anterior pituitary are connected by a portal system.
- The posterior pituitary contains axons that have their cell bodies in the supraoptic and paraventricular nuclei of the hypothalamus.

- Excessive circulating glucocorticoids result in a syndrome characterized by truncal obesity, hypertension, abdominal stria and multiple other signs and symptoms.
- Glucocorticocoid levels may be high as a result of exogenous administration, primary adrenal hypersecretion or hypersecretion due to excess ACTH production.

ADDITIONAL READING

Greenspan FS & Strawler GJ (1997) *Basic and Clinical Endocrinology*, 5th edition. Appleton & Lange, Stanford.

Griffin GE & Ojeda SR (2000) *Textbook of Endocrine Physiology*, 4th edition. Oxford University Press, New York.

Hurley DM & Ho KK (2004) MJA practice essentials – endocrinology. 9: Pituitary disease in adults. *Medical Journal of Austalia* **180**: 419–25.

Kaesoh B (2000) *Endocrine Physiology*. McGraw Hill, New York.

Schuff KG (2003) Issues in the diagnosis of Cushing's syndrome for the primary care physician. *Primary Care* **30**:791–9.

Index

expiratory flow/volume loop 59–60, 63
eyes, puffy 118, *119*

faeces 95
    dark 94
        fatty 77, 79, 80–1, 93
        pale 91, 93, 94
fainting
    in heat stress 142
    in heart disease 67, 68, 69, 70, 73
fatigue, chronic 43–9, 76–82, 118–27,
        153–8
feminization, male 93, 95
ferritin 78, 80
fertility, in spinal cord injury 5, 8
fetal growth and viability, assessment
        37–8, 40
filtration fraction 130
fitness, physical 19, 24, 136, 139–40
    testing 143
fluid balance, in exercise and heat 137–9,
        141–2
fluid replacement
    in anaphylaxis 29
    during exercise 137–9, 141–2
    in haemorrhage 86, 87, 146, 148, 149,
        150
    in metabolic alkalosis 13–14, 15, 16
fluid retention
    in liver disease 92, 93, 95
    in renal disease 51, 52, 53, 56
    see also oedema
folic acid deficiency 79, 80
follicle-stimulating hormone (FSH) 155
food ingestion, before exercise 137, 140
forced expiratory volume in one second
        (FEV1) 19, 24, 58–9, 62–3
forced vital capacity (FVC) 19, 24, 58–9,
        62–3
fractional excretion 130
fructose 79
functional residual capacity (FRC) 58–9,
        62–3
furosemide 53, 55, 56, 135, 148, 150

gamma glutamyl transferase (GGT) 91, 93
gas gangrene 26
gas mixtures, for divers 22, 23, 25–6
gastric acid
    drugs reducing/neutralizing 10, 14
    secretion 10, 14, 15–16
gastric emptying, during exercise 138
gastric glands 11, 14, 15–16

gastric juice 11, **12**
gastric ulcer 16
gastrin 6, 11, 15–16
gastro-colic reflex 6
gastrointestinal tract
    function, in spinal cord injury 2, 6
    hormones 11
    sodium and water absorption 78, 80, *81*
gastro-oesophageal sphincter obstruction
        14
gender differences
    haematocrit 107, 113
    Vo_{2max} 136, 140
Gilbert's disease *92*, 93, 95
glomerular filtration rate (GFR)
    in chronic renal failure 130, 131, 132, 133
    in nephrotic syndrome **51**, 53, 54, 55–6
    factors affecting 51, 55
glomerulonephritis 53, 55, 131
glucocorticoids (corticosteroids) 32, 53,
        64, 157
    see also cortisol
glucose
    ingestion, during exercise 139, 140–2
    plasma
        elevated 98, 102
        fasting 98, 102
    in urine 102
glucose–sodium co-transporter 142
glucose tolerance test 99, 102, 103
glucuronyl-transferase 92, 93, 94, 95
gluten enteropathy *see* coeliac disease
goitre 111–12, 115, 125
Graves' disease 124, 125
growth
    fetal 37–8
    slow in childhood 76–82
growth hormone 154, 156

H1-receptor antagonists 14, 29, 32
H2-receptor antagonists 10, 14
haematocrit (Hct) 76–7, 79, 107
    in blood loss 145, 146, 148
    gender differences 107, 113
    at high altitude 110, 114, 116
    in nephrotic syndrome **51**, 54
haemochromatosis 80
haemoglobin (Hb) concentration 76–7,
        79, 107, 122
    in blood loss 145, 146, 148
    in nephrotic syndrome **51**, 54
haemoglobin saturation *see* oxygen
        saturation

haemophilia 74
haemorrhage 85–89, 145–52
    intracerebral 105
    intrathoracic 85–6, 87, 89
Hashimoto's disease 124
HDL (high-density lipoprotein) 72, 99,
        103
hearing tests 20–1, 25
heart failure 47, 49, 62
    in aortic stenosis 70–1
    at high altitude 111, 116
heart rate
    in anaphylaxis 28, 29, 32
    cardiac filling time at high 140, *141*
    in spinal cord injury 1, 5
    in haemorrhage 83, 86, **87**, 145
    as marker of atrial fibrillation 98, 102
    as marker of atrioventricular block 70,
        73
    maximal, during exercise 136, 140
    reserve 143
    see also bradycardia; tachycardia
heart sounds 68, 72, 74
heat exhaustion 144
heat loss
    prevention, in cold conditions 112–13
    promoting, in hyperthermia 139, 142
heat production, during exercise 143–4
heat stress 139, 142
heat stroke 144
Helicobacter pylori 15, 16, 17
helium 25–6
hemianopsia 99
hemiparesis 97, 99, 100, 105
Henderson–Hasselbalch equation 14–15,
        17, 61
heparin 3, 6, 31
hepatitis 92, 95
high altitude 26, 107–17
high-density lipoprotein (HDL) 72, 99,
        103
histamine 14, 16, 32
H+/K+ ATPase *see* proton pump
hot conditions, acclimatization 141
hydrogen ions (H+; protons)
    in cerebral autoregulation 104
    renal secretion 13, 15, 149
    see also pH
3-hydroxyl-3-methylglutaryl (HMG) CoA
        reductase 100
hyperbaric oxygen 23, 26, 27
hyperbaric physiology 18–27
hypercalcaemia **152**